Health Activism

Foundations and Strategies

Glenn Laverack

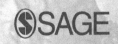

SAGE

Los Angeles | London | New Delhi
Singapore | Washington DC

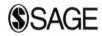

Los Angeles | London | New Delhi
Singapore | Washington DC

SAGE Publications Ltd
1 Oliver's Yard
55 City Road
London EC1Y 1SP

SAGE Publications Inc.
2455 Teller Road
Thousand Oaks, California 91320

SAGE Publications India Pvt Ltd
B 1/I 1 Mohan Cooperative Industrial Area
Mathura Road
New Delhi 110 044

SAGE Publications Asia-Pacific Pte Ltd
3 Church Street
#10-04 Samsung Hub
Singapore 049483

Editor: Alison Poyner
Assistant editor: Emma Milman
Production editor: Katie Forsythe
Copyeditor: Rosemary Morlin
Proofreader: Thea Watson
Marketing manager: Tamara Navaratnam
Cover design: Wendy Scott
Typeset by: C&M Digitals (P) Ltd, Chennai, India
Printed by MPG Books Group, Bodmin, Cornwall

© Glenn Laverack 2013

First published 2013

Library of Congress Control Number: 2012943141

British Library Cataloguing in Publication data

A catalogue record for this book is available from the British Library

ISBN 978-1-4462-4964-2
ISBN 978-1-4462-4965-9 (pbk)

FSC
www.fsc.org   MIX
Paper from
responsible sources
FSC® C018575

Contents

List of figures and boxes

Figures

Boxes

About the author

Glenn Laverack is seen as a world leader in health promotion and empowerment and has had a distinguished Career in public health for more than 25 years working in Europe, Africa, Asia, North America and the Pacific regions. He formerly worked as the Coordinator (Empowerment) at the WHO in Geneva and is presently working at the South Australian Community Health Research Unit, the Southgate Institute, Flinders University. Dr Laverack has a wide range of publications regarding empowerment in international settings including books in English, Russian and German. His range of professional experience in many cross-cultural settings helps to provide a broad insight into empowerment both at the theoretical and practice levels and to find solutions to the causes of social injustice and health inequalities.

Source statement

This book has been written in discussion with many practitioners, academics, researchers and community workers and draws on information from many different contemporary sources. It uses empirical research, case studies and other examples sourced from my own experience, material from the grey literature or systematically collected evidence by others, such as internet sites and web-based data bases, all clearly cited and referenced to indicate the relative strength of the information that is presented or at least to acknowledge its limitations.

Preface

In this book I have defined activism as action on behalf of a cause, action that goes beyond what is conventional or routine, relative to actions used by others in society (Martin, 2007). The 1960s and 1970s was a period of ascendancy for activism both at a theoretical level, championed by thinkers such as Saul Alinsky and Paulo Freire, and by challenges to the existing order though civil protests and disobedience whenever it was perceived to cause an injustice. For a period of time in the mid-1980s to the 1990s, activism was on the decline while practice lagged behind its rhetoric of empowerment and while there was a sense of optimism in the power of the economy and in democracy. But the times changed and more recently there has been a timely revival of health activism.

Driven by global political and economic conditions many governments have pursued a tighter agenda, opting to reduce their responsibility by increasing market choice, transforming national health services into insurance-based health care systems and privatising medical care (Navarro, 2009). For everyday living conditions this has meant cutting pay and jobs, freezing benefits and welfare payments and reducing opportunities for community empowerment (Nathanson and Hopper, 2010). The imbalance in the distribution of power and resources that this has created has contributed to a rise in health inequalities. This is especially the case for those lower down the social gradient (Marmot et al., 2010). Politicians and corporations are unwilling to share power with the marginalised in society, those who have less economic or social protection and are therefore more likely to be affected by their decisions, for example, on changing taxation and the labour market.

Activism is again being used as an expression of public dissatisfaction and as the means to take action against the perpetrators of social injustice and health inequality. This book discusses in detail how health activism has been used in the past and how it can be used in the future as a strategy to help others to take more control of their lives. In particular, the rapidly changing technological environment has enabled activism to take advantage of new developments in communications for better mobilisation to lever access to power and resources. This book offers a revolutionary reorientation of the way we work, of activism as a legitimate approach in the way we deliver health programmes, at a time when innovative ideas in practice are lacking.

Glenn Laverack, Adelaide, Australia

Acknowledgements

I would like to acknowledge the many people with whom I have had the privilege of working and exchanging ideas during the course of writing this book. In particular I would like to thank Cynthia Smith for her insightful comments on the final draft and to Katy Osborne, Toby Freeman, Anna Ziersch, Darlene NcNaughton, Per-Anders Tengland and Janina Curbach for their useful contributions to earlier drafts. My appreciation also to Anne Jones, Nicky Hager, Bob Burton, Simon Chapman, Kathy Barnsley, James O'Brien and Fran Baum for their insights into activism.

Most of all to my family, Elizabeth, Ben, Holly and Rebecca for their unconditional love and support.

1

Foundations of health activism

Activism

Activism is action on behalf of a cause, action that goes beyond what is conventional or routine (Martin, 2007). What constitutes activism depends therefore on what is 'conventional' as any action is relative to others used by individuals, groups and organisations in society. For example, where free speech is respected and protected, posting an email complaining about the government is a routine occurrence. But in an oppressive political system such an action might be seen as subversive and punishable. Likewise, singing in a choir is not activism, but singing as a protest, for example in a prison, can be. Activist actions must therefore go beyond conventional behaviour. However, in practice, organisations employ a combination of both conventional and unconventional strategies and actions to achieve their goals. In systems of representative government, conventional actions include election campaigning, voting, **advocacy** and lobbying politicians. Organisations that use these types of actions are not (and do not consider themselves as) activists because they operate using conventional actions. The circumstances under which activists are willing to use unconventional tactics, whilst others are not, are discussed in this book.

Human rights are central to the manifestos of many political parties. Civil, political, social and cultural human rights such as the freedom of speech and expression, privacy and the right to health, are also fundamental principles in many activist organisations. Activism and conventional politics can therefore operate side-by-side, for example, union activities alongside a Labour Party or environmental movements alongside a Green Party. Activism can be viewed from the local to the global. Local activism is often about protecting the quality of life of a community, such as when residents campaign for better local services or against the location of an industrial development (Strong, 1998). Activism within a country mostly focuses on issues affecting a nation but there is an increasing orientation toward issues crossing national borders at a global level. Local and global forms of activism can be mutually supportive, for example, community opposition to a factory assists, and is assisted by, an environmentalist agenda (Martin, 2007).

Activism has an explicit purpose to help to empower others and this is embodied in actions that are typically energetic, passionate, innovative, and committed. Activism has played a major role in protecting workers from exploitation, protecting the environment, promoting equality for women and opposing racism. However, activism is not necessarily always for a positive cause as the actions of minority groups can oppose human rights and the beliefs of others. To some, an activist is a freedom fighter, to others he/she may be a protagonist, troublemaker, vandal or terrorist. Activists are pragmatic and tend to draw on whatever information is useful for their immediate practical purposes; they want information about a situation and what is effective for dealing with it. Involvement in an activist organisation can begin by attending a public meeting and then by gradually becoming more engaged. Other people become heavily involved in the organisation very quickly but drop out due to other commitments. It is difficult to maintain a high level of involvement, especially as many activists are volunteers and may have a full-time job and a family. Some sorts of activism such as attending a vigil can last for weeks and are difficult for those with other commitments to attend. One of the challenging tasks for organisations is to develop campaigns that allow many people to participate, not just those who have the free time to be able to do so. Someone working on a campaign might spend time listening to the news, reading and sending emails, phoning others, participating in a meeting or writing a grant proposal. 'Frontline action' in which people are participating in support work, usually behind the scenes, is an essential part of what makes activist actions possible. Those involved in behind-the-scenes work, in support of a cause, may call themselves activists, supporters or members of an activist group. Other people who take part may not think of themselves as activists. They are simply doing what is necessary to address a pressing problem. Activist groups run training sessions for their members, but most learning occurs on a person-to-person basis, through direct instruction and learning by doing (Martin, 2007). This can be supplemented by online resources that are freely available on subjects such as community organising, campaigning, and fund raising (Fitzroy Legal Service Inc, 2012). Alternatively, activist organisations may issue their own materials such as general purpose booklets for newly recruited members involved in the campaign on how to organise themselves, where to get information, how to protest, where to find local health care and how to deal with authorities including arrests and police harassment.

Strategies for activism

The types of actions that activist organisations engage in can be broadly subdivided into two categories: indirect and direct actions.

1. Indirect actions are non-violent and conventional and often require a minimum of effort although collectively they can have a dramatic effect. Indirect actions include voting, signing a petition, taking part in a 'virtual (online) sit-in' and sending a letter or email to a person or organisation to protest your cause.

2. For most activists, their focus is on short-term, reactive, direct tactics as their primary, and often only, means of action. Direct actions can become progressively more 'unconventional', from peaceful **protests** to inflicting intentional physical damage to persons and property. Direct action is a form of activity that aims to have a real-time and immediate effect, such as the stopping of work at a construction site that may have broader consequences for people in positions of authority or on future agenda setting.

Direct actions can be further sub-divided into: non-violent and violent actions.

2.1 Non-violent direct actions include protests, **picketing**, vigils, marches, rent strikes, product **boycotts**, withdrawing bank deposits, publicity campaigns and taking legal action.
2.2 Direct violent actions include physical tactics against people or property, placing oneself in a position of manufactured vulnerability to prevent action such as '**digger diving**', squatting in a house detailed for demolition or taking part in a civil disobedience involving the damage of personal property.

Direct action can be symbolic and challenging, sending a message to the general public, and/or to the owners, shareholders, and employees of a specific company, and/or to policymakers, about specific grievances and threats. For example, engaging in direct action that blockaded the roads around the G8 summit in Scotland in 2005 was an example of symbolic direct action, drawing the world's attention to the high levels of anger felt by the anti-globalisation movement. Even though the protests were relatively successful in terms of the amount of disruption to the summit they caused, such direct action would not by itself solve the problems of globalisation, but it did succeed in drawing attention to the key issues (Plows, 2007).

Some organisations use a dual strategic approach: one which is moderate and conventional whilst also using unconventional and more radical tactics. The radical strategy is carried out by individuals or covert **affinity groups**, 'independent' of the organisation, whilst the conventional tactics form the 'official' actions of the organisation. In practice the dynamics of this relationship are often unclear. However, a strategy that employs both conventional tactics such as lobbying and unconventional tactics such as publicity stunts, can have a dramatic influence on public opinion. The environmentalist movement Greenpeace and Code Pink, an international organisation dedicated to uniting women against violence (Code Pink, 2012), have used this approach. The risk is that the unconventional tactics can result in negative publicity and impact on future resource allocation and recruitment to the organisation. Some organisations do not accept donations from governments or corporations and depend instead on contributions from individuals and the assistance from volunteers in order to maintain an independent agenda. The balance between individual autonomy and group responsibility, and the relative importance of means and ends, are therefore often points of contention in using conventional and increasingly violent actions. Tactics vary from country to country and from organisation to organisation and the autonomy exercised by activists and their non-hierarchical structure makes a dual strategic approach both a viable and an attractive option (Martin, 2007).

The range of tactics used by activists can be explained as a dynamic continuum (see Figure 1.1) that progresses from conventional, peaceful tactics to increasingly unconventional, illegal and more violent actions. Some organisations, those that do not fall within the definition of activism, remain on the left-hand side of the continuum and use only conventional tactics. Other organisations, groups and individuals are willing to progress further along the right-hand side of the continuum to engage in unconventional tactics that are disruptive and violent. The continuum is dynamic because organisations can use a variety of tactics that move up and down the continuum, culturally informed and to some extent shaped by local laws. If the use of conventional tactics by an organisation is not successful then it may choose to use more radical tactics further along the continuum as a part of their overall strategy.

Health activism

Health activism is a combination of two key concepts: activism (discussed above) and health. But what do we mean by 'health'? There are many different ways to define and interpret health, each of them leading to different strategies to improve and to gain more control over its determinants. Health's many definitions include the World Health Organization's classic: 'a state of complete physical, mental and social well-being and not merely the absence of disease and infirmity' (World Health Organization, 1948); and the Ottawa Charter's emphasis on it being: 'a resource for everyday life' (World Health Organization, 1986); to the extended Bangkok Charter's qualification of it as; 'a determinant of quality of life … encompassing mental and spiritual well-being' (World Health Organisation, 2005). The important elements of the concept of health that we might take from these definitions are: (1) perception and meaning (health is as much what is experienced as what can be measured), (2) social relations (health is embedded in human **networks** and interactions), (3) capacities/capabilities (health is a product of many intrinsic and extrinsic resources) and (4) physical functioning (health is embodied and not simply imagined) (Laverack, 2009).

Official definitions of health can differ significantly from lay definitions but both are ideal types and in practice coexist and inform one another. Practitioners have embraced a discourse that uses an official definition that goes beyond health care and lifestyle to feelings of well-being. Health is considered to be a means to an end that can be expressed in functional terms as a resource which permits people to lead an individually, socially and economically productive life. However, in practice, public health programming has increasingly been concerned with accountability to funders, effectiveness and value for money (Boutilier, 1993). Budgetary constraints and competition for funding priorities have also had a strong influence on the way in which health has been interpreted. The public health profession has taken the pragmatic view that whatever interpretation of health is used, it must be measurable and accountable, otherwise programmes employing its ideology and strategies will risk being unable to

Attend a community, corporate or government planning meeting. Vote at a local or national election. Lobby a politician or attend a Lobby Day, e-petitions. Create an advocacy group.	Assuming a moral superiority, use moral suasion or soft power by taking/publishing an ethical or philosophical position that is seen as better than another. Send a letter of protest, email or text to a local MP or newspaper.	A product boycott to lever influence with manufacturers. Deliver promotional campaign material house to house.	Peaceful civil protests and demonstrations such as sit-ins, die-ins, picketing, rallies, protest songs, vigils, lock-ins and 'guerrilla camping'. Refusal to pay taxes or bills, rent strikes. Infiltrate a shareholders' meeting or organisation. Take part in strike action, walk-outs, work to rule.	Create a media event such as climbing a public building to deploy a banner, graffiti, deface posters, crop trashing. Engage in an aggressive publicity campaign. Instigate legal action against a person or organisation.	ICT actions including anonymous hacking into another computer, 'Hacktivism', cyberactivism, blogging, viral labeling, virtual sit-ins, circulating a virus package.	Physically alter something to prevent action such as 'spiking' trees with metal pins. Place oneself in a position of manufactured vulnerability such as occupying a tunnel under a road, squatting in a house for demolition, 'digger diving', 'lock-ons'. Take part in a riot with the intention to carry out physical damage on property or persons.

Conventional and indirect   **Unconventional and direct**

Figure 1.1 Continuum of activist actions

justify their economic and quantifiable effectiveness. This being the case, the measurement of health has focused on the bio-medical approach that is concerned with demonstrating a relationship between a health status measure and a behaviour such as smoking or a condition such as morbidity and mortality. The boundaries for practice and discourse have consequently been defined by the interpretations of illness and disease rather than by the way in which most people generally view their own health.

The bio-medical model evolved as a result of scientific discoveries and technological advances in the eighteenth and nineteenth centuries and this led to a greater understanding of the structure and functioning of the human body. As knowledge and understanding increased, health took on an increasingly mechanistic meaning. The body was viewed as a machine that needed to be repaired. A professional split between the body and mind developed, the body and its physical illnesses were the responsibility of physicians while psychologists and psychiatrists looked after the psyche and its abnormalities. However, the focus remained on the external causes of ill health and was reinforced by the constant threat of disease and death from epidemics such as polio and scarlet fever (Laverack, 2009). The biomedical era continued to dominate until the 1960s and 1970s, when the growing costs of publicly funded health care collided with one of capitalism's cyclical crises of too much supply, too little demand and a declining rate of profit. This led to market pressures on the state to lessen taxation and liberalise the economy, which in turn fuelled government interest to find ways to reduce the fiscal pressure of rising medical care costs. At the same time, the 'epidemiological transition' in high-income countries was complete: few infectious diseases remained as threats and chronic degenerative illnesses (heart disease, cancer, autoimmune disorders) had become the major causes of morbidity and mortality. These chronic diseases involve the interplay of different behavioural risk factors over time such as smoking, lack of exercise and a poor diet, and have become synonymous with a 'healthy lifestyle'. The search for genetic explanation had yet to commence and few were discussing the role poverty or hazardous environments played in creating disease. Health education to modify unhealthy behaviours became the principal public health intervention, slowly expanding to a broader policy focus to influence the economic and cultural forces that pattern unhealthy behaviours. As with the biomedical approach, however, there was little room for concerns with **empowerment** and activism and the tendency of practice was to focus on individuals in ways that became victim-blaming (Labonté and Penfold, 1981). The confluence of state interests in medical cost containment, the rise of chronic disease with more scope for prevention and the emergence of powerful new **social movements** (feminism, **environmentalism**, the New Left, civil rights), nonetheless created fertile ground for a 'new' public health embrace of 'old' public health activism.

Peter Aggleton (1991), a commentator on public health issues, divides the official interpretations of health into two main types: those which define health negatively, and those which adopt a more positive stance. There are two main ways of viewing health negatively. The first equates with the absence of disease or bodily abnormality, the second with the absence of illness or the feelings of anxiety, pain or distress that may or may not accompany the disease. Aggleton points to the importance of recognising that some people may be diseased without knowing it. People are unaware of their illnesses until they start to suffer pain and discomfort, when the person is said to be ill. Negative definitions of health emphasise the absence of disease or illness and are the basis for the medical model. A number of problems have been raised concerning the negative definition of health. In particular, the notion of pathology implies that certain universal 'norms' exist against which an individual can be assessed when making a judgment as to whether or not they are healthy. This assumes that such standards actually exist in human anatomy and physiology. The way in which people interpret the meaning of their own health is a personal and sometimes unique experience. Health is a subjective concept and its interpretation is relative to the environment and culture in which people find themselves. Health can mean different things to different people. Many people define health in functional terms by their ability to carry out certain roles and responsibilities rather than the absence of disease. People may be willing to bear the discomfort and pain of an illness because it does not outweigh the inconvenience, loss of control or financial cost of having the condition treated (Laverack, 2009). But on a day-to-day basis most people are not concerned if their health is perfect and instead are concerned with the trade-offs they have to make in order to live their lives. Cohen and Henderson (1991) cite examples of people who are diseased or ill and yet still perceive themselves as being healthy and willing to bear the discomfort and pain of an illness because it does not outweigh the inconvenience, loss of control or financial cost of having the condition treated. People are willing to make certain 'trade-offs' such as leading a stressful lifestyle, doing less exercise, smoking or drinking alcohol, in deciding what they need, or want to do, to live life but at the same time experience being healthy. However, there are situations in which people feel that even given their own personal 'trade-offs' that they are prevented from leading a healthy life because of, for example, the lack of opportunity or an injustice.

People may be sure about what they want but are often less certain about the means to achieve it, especially how to gain access to political influence and resources. Under such situations, people are motivated to empower themselves in order to achieve what they need and want. To become empowered involves a process by which people gain more control over the decisions and resources that influence their lives and health. Community empowerment builds from the individual to the group to a wider collective and embodies the intention, as does health activism, to bring about social, political and economic change for improvements in peoples' lives. Empowerment and health activism also share the same sense of struggle and liberation that is bound in the process of gaining power. Power cannot be given but must be gained or seized by those who want it from those who hold it, often those who are in authority. In recent decades, activism has emerged as an effective way for those without great financial resources or political **leverage** to influence the public debate on health issues such as better housing, better health care, more services for people with HIV and stronger oversight of the tobacco industry (Freudenberg et al., 2011). In simple terms, health activism involves a challenge to the existing order whenever it is perceived to influence people's health negatively or has led to an injustice or an inequity. The tactics of health activism have continued to evolve along with political opportunity and developments in culture and technology. Mobile phone messaging and the internet, for example, are now extensively used in activism to organise rallies and to carry out online tactics (discussed in Chapter 6). Health activism also continues to raise new issues including sexual harassment, bullying, and domestic violence by campaigning about them and by developing techniques to address the inequities that these issues create (Plows, 2007).

Women and activism

Women have historically come together to form partnerships with one another to share knowledge. For example, the feminist movement supported activism through a network of individuals and groups, has fostered learning about tactics, and has offered an understanding of the problem of patriarchy through the sharing of experiences (Pakulski, 1991). The role of feminism is discussed extensively elsewhere in the literature and is not intended to be a core part of this chapter. However, it is worthwhile stating that women's activism has been a key movement in relation to health and has addressed a range of issues including reproductive and sexual health, maternal health, child care, the menopause, breast and ovarian cancer, osteoporosis and safety from domestic violence (Worsham, 2007).

Code Pink, for example, is an international organisation dedicated to uniting women against international and domestic violence. The group follows feminist ideals and advocates open and respectful communication and creative unconventional tactics. Using the internet, media coverage, pop culture, and protests, Code Pink uses 'enjoyable' activism, including die-ins and teach-ins, offering highly visual events that attract media attention. Code Pink has also created a number of partnerships with other organisations supporting peace and justice (Code Pink, 2012).

'Mothers against drunk driving' (MADD), founded by a mother whose daughter was killed by a drunk driver, is a non-profit organisation in the United States that seeks to stop drunk driving, support those affected by drunk driving, prevent underage drinking and to lobby for stricter alcohol policy. MADD is opposed to the criminal act of drunk driving, not individuals, and to support the victims of violent crime. Similar **pressure groups** have also developed in reaction to a range of issues about which mothers feel strongly and that have affected their lives, for example, 'Mothers against violence', 'Mothers against guns', 'Mothers against drugs' and 'Mothers against knives'. MADD actions include:

- education (about the dangers of drunk driving), advocacy and victim assistance;
- strict policy in a variety of areas including blood alcohol level, mandatory jail sentences, treatment for alcoholism and ignition interlock devices;
- helping victims of drunk driving (this includes family members and other loved ones of both innocent victims and guilty impaired drivers);
- maintaining the minimum legal drinking age at 21 years.

MADD promotes the use of victim impact panels (VIPs), in which judges require offenders to hear victims or relatives of victims of drunk driving crashes relate their experiences. The presentations are often emotional, detailed, and graphic, and focus on the tragic negative consequences of alcohol-related crashes (MADD, 2012).

Women's health activism is advocacy for and a commitment to non-discrimination and informed consent in health because women often have not had the power to control and make decisions about their own bodies. The women's health movement has always striven for a woman's right to choose and be informed of her health options in collaboration with others. For example, the first birth-control pill was developed by men and tested on Puerto Rican women in the 1950s and became a prescription drug in 1960. Though it was initially met with enthusiasm, investigations by women's health activists, such as Barbara Seaman (1935–2008), exposed the risks of such a highly hormonal, and largely untested, fertility regimen and, more significantly, exposed the lack of information shared with women as patients, who took the pill every day. The pill remains a popular method of contraception, but because of health activism, women have increased access to information about medical treatment and are no longer expected to take instructions on the choice of contraception from medical professionals without question (Daly, 2007).

Social justice, equity and health inequity

Health activism and social justice evolved as important ideologies in the mid-nineteenth century. In particular, the period around 1848 was pivotal because a number of key popular uprisings and social movements were pursuing an agenda of social justice, including the socialist and trade union movements in Europe, the anti-slavery and women's rights movements in the USA, and resistance to imperialism in India. In 1848 Europe saw the revolution in France and the first public health act in Britain (Krieger and Birn, 1998). The political liberalism of the Victorian period in the UK led to the creation of many pressure groups, such as the Health of Towns Association, with a concern for equity and social justice. The Association existed only briefly between 1844 and 1849 and promoted sanitary reform in rapidly growing areas of urban industrialisation. The Association organised regional interest groups, lectures and published the 'journal of public health' to raise awareness amongst professional groups and to lobby opinion leaders. These pressure groups helped key public health reformers, such as Edwin Chadwick (see Chapter 7), to achieve their aim of bringing in the Public Health Act 1848 and to be more active in mobilising the middle classes who in turn had an influence on the press and on the government (Berridge, 2007). These early pressure groups are an example of the combination of science and activism and a period that through both influential reformers and political action resulted in the government passing key public health legislation (Baggott, 2000). The temperance movement differed from the Health of Towns Association in the strategy it used to oppose the drinking of spirits and beer to the point of total abstinence. The strategy concentrated on 'moral suasion', on the establishment of a mass movement of mostly working men to take a 'pledge' to cease from the use of alcohol. Moral suasion is the act of trying to use moral principles to influence individuals and groups to change their practices, beliefs and actions. The strategy focused on targeting individual behaviour change rather than structural change or government intervention. The movement offered support through a set of self-help groups and worked across the classes in society advocating for a sober workforce as well as for 'teetotallers' everywhere (Berridge, 2007).

A contrasting issue but a similar approach concerns foot-binding that was universal where practiced in China, painful and dangerous and afflicted Chinese women for a millennium. And yet this practice ended, for the most part, in a single generation. The natural-foot movement was championed by liberal modernisers and women's rights advocates and developed in the years of change culminating in the revolution of 1911. Reform and urban economic development were part of modernisation and migration from the countryside consequently provided alternative opportunities of support for women strengthening their independence and bargaining power. The pivotal innovation was also moral suasion by forming **alliances**, called 'pledge associations', of parents who pledged not to foot-bind their daughters nor let their sons marry foot-bound women (Mackie, 1996) as moral principles for the basis of individual behaviour change.

Two major theories on social justice differ in their emphasis on means or ends: equality of opportunity or equality of outcome. The first, and politically dominant, theory holds to the importance of ensuring that everyone 'plays by the same rules' and that there is no discrimination. Fairness is judged by equality in process. The second, and politically challenging, theory holds to the importance of ensuring that rules work to minimise preventable differences in outcomes between the players. It discriminates positively in favour of those groups who start the 'game' of social and economic life with fewer resources since equal rules for unequal players will always produce unequal results. While fairness in process is important, concerns with preventable differences in health outcomes align themselves ethically more closely to the second theory of justice (Labonté, 2000; Laverack, 2004). Equity, as applied to health, is a normative judgment of what is fair. It differs from equality, a measure of 'sameness', although the terms are often used interchangeably, where health inequality has become synonymous with health inequity (Braveman and Gruskin, 2003). This is particularly so in the UK, where health inequality has become synonymous with health inequity.

In stricter terms, a health inequity is a difference (an inequality) in health that is significant in size and number of people affected, preventable through policy or other interventions and not an effect of freely-chosen risk. A major concern is social inequities that reside in the structures of society, creating systematic differences in health outcomes between different population groups. Examples of these include: gender differences that arise from patriarchal norms or discrimination; class differences that arise from inequalities in wealth, power and ownership/control of capital and geographic differences that arise from higher exposures to risk or less access to remediable care or preventive resources. This is a link between individual control and health that has been demonstrated in several studies including (Everson et al., 1997) a study of Finnish middle-aged white males concluding that stress induced from job demands and feelings of a lack of control was the strongest predictor of arterial heart disease. A review of heart health inequalities in Canada found that people who experience low income, less control in their lives and at work and who had a poor education are more likely to experience morbidity and mortality. In other words, the higher one's position in the workplace or society, one's power (control), wealth and status, the better one's health and sense of self-esteem (Labonté, 1993).

Internationally, the need for social justice in the challenge to improve health has become the subject of professional discourse through key documents and international meetings, for example, the international conference on primary health care in Alma Ata (World Health Organization, 1978) in 1978 endorsed 'health for all' and strongly affirmed the WHO's positive definition of health (World Health Organization, 1986), noting that it was a fundamental human right. Since the early 1980s, there has also been an increased awareness of growing inequalities in health status between different social groups and of the narrowness of the focus on individual behaviour that ignored the psychosocial and physical environments, community and culture. The individualistic nature of public-health education campaigns did not recognise the social and environmental contexts in which personal behaviours are embedded and which were important health determinants. Another significant factor was the maturing of many pressure groups and social movements such as the environmentalists and the human rights movements, who challenged the notion of the medical and behavioural approaches to health and raised concerns for social justice and environmental sustainability (Freeman, 1983). The role of the social movements is discussed in Chapter 2.

It is now, more than ever, recognised that the key to addressing inequalities in health is through the redistribution of power and by transforming unequal power relationships within and between societies. Health inequity in the conditions of daily living is shaped by deep social structures and processes, is systematic and can be enhanced by social norms and government policies that tolerate or actually promote unfair distribution of and access to power, wealth and other necessary social resources (World Health Organization, 2008).

Next, I discuss the different forms of power and how these can have a significant influence on people's level of control over their lives and health.

Power

The radical perspective

An increase in political instability combined with forms of government dominated by elite interests has led to the oppression of human rights in some countries. Under these circumstances, people can feel that social justice in society does not exist and when they lose their basic rights, for example, to protest or to a fair voting and legal system, they may use the only resource they have, the capacity to cause trouble. The forms of direct action that they can use include riots, insurgency and violence, or the threat of violence. The fear that they create and the reaction of those in power become the basis for political influence. This is a risky option because it relies on dramatic social and political change and so

the protesters must maximise their efforts to succeed and push for full concessions in return for a cease to the disruptions. This is the radical perspective.
Frances Fox Piven and Richard Cloward (1977), two influential American social
reformers, point out that historically the radical perspective has given rise to
examples of radical change. In circumstances in which people believe they have
nothing to lose, for example, when they have no employment, no property or
have no hope for the future, then it is a logical 'make or break' option. Direct
action such as witnessed in the Arab Spring in North Africa (see Box 1.1), for
example, started from the actions of one person and drew upon civil unrest to
create radical social and political change.

Box 1.1   The Arab Spring

The Arab Spring is a revolutionary movement that swept across the Arab world
beginning on Saturday 18 December 2010 in Tunisia, acting as a catalyst for
subsequent activist actions in Egypt, Libya, Syria and the Yemen. In Tunisia, the
actions of one man, a vegetable seller (Mohamed Bouazizi), sparked the
revolution by setting himself alight after his goods were confiscated by police.
The people who knew Bouazizi, his friends, family and neighbours, quickly
assembled at the government offices and a protest began. People in the crowd
took pictures and videos that were posted on Facebook or sent to Al-Jazeera,
the Arabic-language television network. When the Tunisian government blocked
the internet, the demonstrators used their mobile phones to send messages
and images. The Arab Spring's mass strategy involved strikes, demonstrations,
marches and rallies, as well as the use of media advocacy. **Internet activism**
involving the use of Facebook and Twitter were used to organise and to
communicate to people across the region and across the world. These actions
were largely politically driven as indicated in the slogan of the demonstrators
'the people want to bring down the regime'. However, other inequities
contributing to the civil unrest included human rights violations, unemployment,
poverty, dictatorship, increasing food prices and corruption within government.
A rising tension between an aspiring educated young population and a lack of
reform by the government also underlay the civil unrest that soon spread
across the region resulting in the destruction of property, deaths and, in some
cases, the overthrow of government, as was the case in Libya (Abulof, 2011;
Khalaf, 2011).

In oppressive social and political circumstances, radical action is sometimes the
most effective means of utilising the limited resources available to the
marginalised in society. This 'strategy of tension' is a concept of manipulation,
change and control of public opinion using tactics of fear, propaganda and mass
protests. Some groups may even embark on a process that uses tactics based on
coordinated indiscriminate attacks, targeting innocent people not involved in the

issue, sometimes with an apparent disregard for human life. Radical action can have a negative impact on people's lives when they are affected by a process that can promote violence and fear. We live in a world in which access to resources and decisions are limited and competing interests struggle to gain control. The reality is that this includes competition between groups that strive to bring about social and political change and that are willing to use extreme strategies.

Hard power

The common interpretation of **hard power** is as power-over individuals and groups, '... the capacity of some persons to produce intended and foreseen effects on others' (Wrong, 1988: 2). The German social scientist, Max Weber (1947: 152), offers a similar definition of power as 'the probability that one actor within a social relationship will be in a position to carry out his own will despite resistance'. Weber identifies two forms of power which he closely links to conflict, one where conflict is absent and the other where the resistance of others must be overcome. Richard Adams (1977: 387) extends the idea of power further by vesting it in both individuals and social groups, as '... the ability of a person or social unit to influence the conduct and decision making of another through the control over energetic forms in the latter's environment ...'. These interpretations are all variations on how power is commonly referenced in the social science literature: one person having influence and mastery over another. To exercise choice is the simplest form of power. This may involve the trivial choices of everyday life or the more critical choices and decisions which influence health. To the extent our personal choices constrain those of others, it becomes an exercise of power-over. For example, people with the ability to control decisions at the political and economic level condition and constrain the ability of other people to exercise control or choice at the individual and group levels. Sometimes we willingly accord people this 'higher' level ability, such as when legislation is passed to prevent or punish people, to protect the health of others (Laverack, 2004).

Soft power

In contrast to hard power, **soft power** is the ability to obtain what one wants through indirect and long-term actions such as co-option and attraction. The purpose is to persuade others to voluntarily do what you want them to do, avoiding conflict and tension. The primary currencies of soft power are values, culture, policies and institutions, agenda control and the extent to which these are able to attract or repel others to 'want what you want' (Gallarotti, 2011). Soft power is a descriptive rather than a normative concept, one that has not been theoretically well developed and like any form of power, can be wielded for good or bad purposes. Soft power is not merely non-traditional forces such as cultural and commercial goods, as this confuses the resources that may produce the desired behaviour. The phrase 'you are either with us or against us' is an exercise in soft power, since no explicit threat is included. However, rationalists would argue that this is an 'implied threat' and that direct economic or military sanctions would likely follow from being 'against us'. The success of soft power can depend on one person's reputation as well as on the flow of information. Media is regularly identified as a source of soft power, as is the spread of a national language, or a particular set of normative values. Because soft power has appeared as an alternative to hard power, it is often embraced by ethically-minded scholars and policymakers, but has been criticised as being ineffective and too difficult to distinguish from the effects of other factors. The difference between soft and hard power is that the latter achieves compliance through more direct and coercive methods and by compelling others to do what you want them to do, whether they want to do it or not. An example is health insurance where individuals often choose protection against disease, accidents and illnesses to guarantee treatment and recovery. It may be possible to receive protection without insurance, consistent with soft power, from relatives, friends or from a welfare system (if it exists). But these are not guaranteed options for recovery in the same way that health insurance (hard power) offers the individual through compensation (Gallarotti, 2011). Another example is 'moral suasion', the use of moral principles to influence individuals and groups to change their practices, beliefs and actions. The person or organisation presents a position of moral superiority by taking an ethical or philosophical stance on an issue such as human rights thereby persuading others, through their soft power, to join them (Berridge, 2007).

Three faces of hard power

Philosopher Thomas Wartenberg (1990) described the two-faced nature of hard power: power-to, or our abilities to do or accomplish something by ourselves; and power-over, or the ability to affect the actions or ideas of others despite their resistance. Starhawk (1990) takes the concept of power-to further and subdivides it into: power-from-within, or one's personal power; and power-with, in which power-over increases other people's power-from-within, rather than to dominate or exploit them. To better understand how hard power is exercised in both a positive (the sharing of control with others) and a negative manner (the use of control to exert influence over others against their will), it is helpful to consider three of its simplest forms: 'power-from-within', 'power-over', and 'power-with.'

Power-from-within

Power-from-within can be described as an experience of 'self', a personal power or some inner sense of integrity or 'truth' (Labonté, 1996). Others argue that power-from-within is gained from philosophical, religious and spiritual sources (Morriss, 1987; Wartenberg, 1990). Power-from-within is also known as individual, personal or psychological empowerment and the many definitions of this concept, developed in the field of psychology in Westernised countries, describe it as gaining (a sense of) control over one's life (Rissel, 1994). Starhawk's (1990: 10) description of power-from-within is similar; she likens it to '... our sense of mastery we develop as young children ...', but also to something deeper '... our sense of bonding with other human beings, and with the environment'. The goal is to increase feelings of value and a sense of individual mastery and to increase the notion of 'self'. Power-from-within is not concerned with access to or control over resources. Individuals can therefore become more powerful from within and do not necessarily have to accumulate power as money, or status or authority.

Power-over

Power-over describes social relationships in which one party is made to do what another party wishes them to, despite their resistance and even if it may not be in their best interests. Starhawk (1990: 9) describes power-over in its clearest form as '... the power of the prison guard, of the gun, power that is ultimately backed by force'. The exercise of power-over does not always have to be negative. State legislation to control the spread of diseases, to impose fines for unhealthy behaviour such as smoking in a public place, or even to redistribute market income to prevent poverty, are all examples of what we consider 'healthy' power-over. Power-over can take different forms depending on how it is used to exert control or to influence others. Many writers settle on three functionally distinct operations of power-over: dominance, or the direct power to control people's choices, usually by force or its threat; exploitation, or the indirect power to control people's choices through economic relations, in which those who control capital (primarily money) also have control over those who do not; and hegemony, or the ability of a dominant group to control the actions and behaviours of others by intense persuasion (Wrong, 1988).

Hegemonic power is that form of power-over that is invisible and internalised such that it is structured into our everyday lives and taken for granted (Foucault, 1979). To Foucault, a prominent theorist and commentator on power, the only form of resistance to hegemonic power was a concealment of one's life from those in authority. For example, the hidden actions of a single mother living in poor housing hiding a messy room or her sick child from a health visitor (Bloor and McIntosh, 1990). Persons living in conditions of hegemonic power-over, of oppression and exploitation, internalise these conditions as being their personal responsibility. This internalisation increases their own self-blame and decreases their self-esteem. This internalisation can lead to false consciousness, a failing to utilise the power one has and failing to acquire powers that one can acquire (Morriss, 1987). Hegemonic power-over is inherently unhealthy, because it shuts down critical thinking, public debate and the possibility of change. One of the subtle ways in which health practitioners participate in hegemonic power-over is when they continually impose their ideas of what are important problems without listening to what others think are important.

The rise of the medical profession has been successful in maintaining its position of dominance within the health institutional hierarchy by controlling access to health care delivery. This has been termed the 'hegemony of the medical profession'. The medical profession has formed itself as a powerful professional pressure group. This manifests itself both as a collective workforce and through key associations, for example in the UK, the British Medical Association and the Royal Colleges. The medical profession, although not a complete monopoly because of the growth of other health professions, has been granted considerable control to maintain self-regulation and clinical autonomy in their work. In fact, the dominance of the medical profession has been blamed for the historical subordination of the nursing profession and a key challenge to nurse empower-ment (Kendall, 1998). Much of the power-over held by the medical profession is also supported by the public who expect confidentiality in the special relation-ship that they hold with their personal doctor. The medical profession is also dependent on various alliances with other health professionals, the government, the private sector, science and activists in civil society. The medical profession has been careful to create an alignment between professional and public interests and its position further strengthened by an increase in the legitimacy of medical knowledge, urbanisation, the expansion of health insurance and the growth of institutional settings such as hospitals as centres for 'professional excellence' (Turner and Samson, 1995).

An example of the early resistance to the dominance of the medical profession is the natural childbirth movement, featured in Box 1.2 below.

Box 1.2 The natural childbirth movement

The natural childbirth movement took a distinctively political turn in the 1960s and 1970s emerging as a response to the common use of drugs and invasive medical procedures during childbirth. The movement resisted the dominance of the medical profession in regard to its support for medicalised childbirth because of concerns about maternal and infant health. Women and feminists struggled for control over their bodies during childbirth and described the health care system as a patriarchal institution that reproduced male physicians' dominant position over labouring women. For some, taking control of childbirth was a step towards women controlling their own lives. Meanwhile, the growing alternative birthing movement rejected technological birthing and while legal and medical resistance to the natural childbirth movement remains, more women are choosing home births, midwives, or birthing centres. Some hospitals have changed rigid rules and provide women with more natural birthing options. There are also numerous organisations, meet-up groups, books, and magazines dedicated to natural childbirth with some of its principles being incorporated into mainstream medicine (Metoyer, 2007).

Power-with

Power-with describes a different set of social relationships, in which power-over is deliberately used to increase other people's power-from-within, rather than to dominate or exploit them. Power-over transforms to power-with only when it has effectively reached its end, when the submissive person in the relationship has accrued enough power-from-within to exercise his or her own choices and decisions. Western feminist theory also supports the concept of power-with in that the greater the development of each individual the more able, effective and less dependent on others they become (Swift and Levin, 1987). Feminist theory holds that even in the most male-dominated, power-over society, women have power, the power-from-within, and they do have special skills and inner strengths that have enabled them to act in invaluable ways (Wartenberg, 1990). Once one has accepted this, the argument that people can both have and lack power-over in society can be seen to contain an important insight. Power-over becomes a decentred notion: a person may hold a great deal of authority in one aspect of their life but possess very little in other aspects of it. An immigrant may hold the position of a leader within their own community, but within the workplace in their adopted country may have only a low-paying menial job with little responsibility and may be considered a second-class citizen by some of their colleagues. The first challenge in these situations is to strengthen an individual's power-from-within, partly by identifying their own sources of power-over and partly by giving them ways to find the solutions to their concerns. The second challenge in these situations is to work with the person to use one's professional power-over to transform to power-with.

Starhawk (1990: 10) identifies the source of power-with as '... the willingness of others to listen to our ideas'. The person with the power-over chooses not to command or exert control, but to suggest and to begin a discussion that will increase the other's sense of power-from-within. With respect to some facets of community members' lives, health practitioners may have knowledge and resources useful to them and may give priority to communities that are relatively powerless. Rather than a simple transfer of resources and information, then, the professional relationship involves an offering of advice and strategies to develop both the psychological empowerment (self-esteem and self-confidence) of individuals and the collective empowerment of communities.

The transformative use of power-over demands a great deal of self-vigilance and self-discipline by all persons in the relationship, but in particular by the initially more dominant person, often the practitioner. Otherwise, the relationship can remain as power-over, for example, legitimate or expert power that does not acknowledge that others in the relationship may have their own expertise can lead to a patronising inducement of dependency. Linden (1994) suggests that the doctor and patient relationship is unequal where all competence is considered to belong to one party, often between a male 'expert' and a female patient. Thus the woman voluntarily surrenders to the unspoken claim of medical (expert) power. The doctor has a monopoly of knowledge even though that knowledge concerns the patient's own body. Medicalisation works within the frame of this double power relation, differences of knowledge and gender. The attributes of health are viewed as an individual 'case' and the diagnosis is made on that basis. Thus the medical model serves to protect the legitimate and expert power of the doctor.

Powerlessness

Powerlessness, or the absence of power, whether imagined or real can be an individual concept with the expectancy that the behaviour of a person cannot determine the outcomes they seek. Powerlessness is viewed as a continuous interaction between the person and his/her environment. It combines an attitude of self-blame, a sense of generalised distrust, a feeling of alienation from resources for social influence, an experience of disenfranchisement and economic vulnerability, and a sense of hopelessness in socio-political struggle (Kieffer, 1984). Powerlessness may also be viewed as a result of the passive acceptance of oppressive cultural 'givens', or the surrender to a 'culture of silence' (Freire, 1973). Paulo Freire believed that the individual becomes powerless in assuming the role of 'object' acted upon by the environment, rather than the 'subject' acting in and on the world. As such, the individual alienates himself/herself from participation in the construction of social reality (Wallerstein, 1992). The powerless often experience little leverage on the events and conditions that impinge on their existence, either directly or through access to resources that guarantee survival, decrease discomfort, and enable change and betterment in one's life (Kroeker, 1995). Rather than begin their work from the perspective that people who are, in general terms, 'relatively' economically and politically powerless, health practitioners need to look for, and work from, areas in peoples' lives in which they are 'relatively' powerful. The challenge is to assist individuals to organise themselves to increase their collective exercise of power-over.

Empowerment

Empowerment in the broadest sense is '... the process by which disadvantaged people work together to increase control over events that determine their lives' (Werner, 1988). Most definitions of empowerment give the term a similarly positive value, and have been largely developed in industrialised countries in the areas of neighbourhood empowerment and community mental health (Rappaport, 1987; Swift and Levin, 1987). These definitions embody the notion that empowerment must come from within an individual, group or community and cannot be given to them. The over-use and misuse of the term has led to it having a lesser significance and a diminished meaning. But it is through collective or community empowerment that people are able to achieve the broader social and political change that is necessary to improve their lives and health. To provide clarity to this concept it is useful to consider the different levels of community empowerment. Christopher Rissel (1994) includes a heightened or increased level of psychological empowerment as a part of community empowerment. He also argues that community empowerment includes '... a political action component in which members have actively participated, and the achievement of some redistribution of resources or decision making favourable to the community or group in question'. Barbara Israel and her colleagues (1994) similarly identify psychological and political action as two levels of community empowerment, but include a third, and intermediary level between them, that of organisational empowerment. Their analysis of this level draws heavily from democratic management theory. An empowered organisation is one that is democratically managed: its members share information and control over decisions and are involved in the design, implementation and control of efforts toward goals defined by group consensus. It is an essential link between empowered individuals and effective political action and is similar to the structure of many activist organisations such as pressure groups and social movements.

Community empowerment includes personal (psychological) empowerment, organisational empowerment and broader social and political changes and is both an individual and group phenomena. It is a dynamic process involving continual shifts in personal empowerment (power-from-within) and changes in power-over relations between different social groups and decision makers in the broader society. Community empowerment as an outcome can vary, for example, as a redistribution of resources (Rappaport, 1984), a decrease in individuals' or groups' powerlessness (Kieffer, 1984) or success in achieving a programme's goals (Purdey et al., 1994). But it is as a process that it is most consistently viewed in the literature, for example, '... a social-action process that promotes participation of people, organisations and communities towards the goals of increased individual and community control, political efficacy, improved quality of life and social justice' (Wallerstein, 1992). As a process, community empowerment is best considered as a continuum representing progressively more organised and broadly-based forms of collective action. The continuum model of community empowerment is discussed in more detail in Chapter 4.

Next, in Chapter 2, I discuss how international social movements, pressure groups and advocacy groups apply the foundations of activism to their work and provide an analysis of the important lessons that can be learnt from their international strategies of what works and what does not work in practice.

2

International experiences of activism

The role of social movements

A social movement can be defined as a sustained and organised public effort targeting authorities that can use both conventional and unconventional strategies to achieve its goals (Tilly, 2004). Criteria to assess whether a social mobilisation meets the requirements to be called a 'movement' have been developed and include:

- the presence of articulated grievances;
- policy goals;
- access to human and financial resources;
- sustained activities to meet these goals;
- leadership;
- participants with a shared worldview and identity. (Freudenberg et al., 2011)

Some of these criteria can also be applied to pressure and advocacy groups. What makes a social movement different is its ability to go beyond the influence of its participant and resource base, to maintain an ideology irrespective of membership, function and organisational structure. To do this, a movement must have 'deep social roots' and this is the defining characteristic that differentiates a movement from the many other action orientated organisations.

One major division in regard to the nature of social movements has been between the views of structural conflict and those that interpret movements as a normal part of change in society. The diversity of theoretical and ideological allegiances have popularly viewed social movements in Westernised countries along three schemata; Resource Mobilisation Theory (RMT), popular with American researchers taking an economic rationalism view, Action Identity Theory (AIT) and New Social Movement Theory (NSMT), popular with European researchers and based on Marxist and Durkheimian traditions. The French sociologist, Émile Durkheim (1858–1917), was concerned primarily with how societies could maintain their integrity and coherence when factors, including shared religious and ethnic background, could no longer be assumed. Durkheim wrote much about the effect of laws, religion, education and other forces on civil society and how social structures influenced, for example, the rate of suicide (Craig and Calhoun, 2002).

It is the emancipatory discourse of the NSMT that is shared by health activists and provides an important context for their actions in several ways:

- They constitute a network of individuals and groups that is a source of communication, advice, and inspiration.
- They provide a learning environment, with activists drawing on the experience of other groups to find out what works.
- They provide a framework that develops out of the experience of activists, combined with the ideas of writers and leaders, some who are part of the movement and some who are largely independent of it. (Pakulski, 1991)

Social movements, in Westernised countries in particular, have been described as leaderless disorganisations, comprising fluid, shifting, autonomous groups and networks that operate independently. In fact a deliberate focus on disorganisation could also be seen as the avoidance of hierarchical power relations and an emphasis on autonomy. Social movements can be also seen as rational actors that are generally reactive, in that they tend to form, and mobilise, in response to specific events and issues. Alternatively, established social movements can start to develop strategies as they build up capacity over time, as previous mobilisation predisposes them to identify other issues that they see as related to their cause (Plows, 2007). However, most analysts believe it is important that social movements do have a structure and a pattern of inter-relations between individuals and groups. This pattern evolves through a process of mobilisation, participation and organisation. Formal social movements may possess bureaucratic procedures but they do not operate from within bureaucracies. New social movements exist within civil society, developed by the people, against dominant structures and ideologies held by those in authority (Pakulski, 1991).

New social movements are not solely concerned with structural revolution or reform but more with cultural and expressive objectives based on the formation of an identity. Identity is created not simply through the existence of a social movement but also through action within the movement (Melucci, 1985). New social movements tend to attract people with a professional and educated background as well as some type of negative experience in regard, for example, to treatment or health care (Allsop et al., 2004). The identity is shared by all its members and it is the process of internal action and negotiation that connects and bonds them through social relationships. The main purpose of the 'new' movements is their transformation of values and change, for example, in the nature of health care and social services, rather than a radical restructuring.

Involvement in a movement can result in marked differences between activist and non-activist members. For example, for those living with HIV/AIDS, members of movements had better coping skills and preferences, knowledge of HIV-treatment and social network integration. The AIDS coalition to unleash power (Act-up) understood this influence and was dedicated to promoting the health and welfare of individuals with HIV/AIDS. Act-up helped people to enhance their ability as individuals to make informed choices about personal health care and HIV/AIDS treatments (Brashers et al., 2002). Involvement in a social movement can also have direct benefits to one's health compared to not participating in a social movement, as shown in Box 2.1 below, featuring the Movimento dos Trabalhadores Rurais Sem Terra.

Box 2.1   Movimento dos Trabalhadores Rurais Sem Terra

In Brazil, 45 per cent of agricultural land is held by around 1 per cent of landowners, while around 50 per cent of proprietors together own only roughly 2 per cent of all arable land. About 31 million Brazilians (18.8 per cent of the total population) live in the countryside. These people, known as *agregados*, are extremely poor and suffer high rates of many psychosocial, educational and health problems. In 1984, landless families organised themselves into the Movimento dos Trabalhadores Rurais Sem Terra (MST), or Movement of Landless Rural Workers. MST is probably the largest social movement in Latin America, with around 1.5 million members. Its fundamental success has been the increasing number of landless families being allocated their own piece of land, rising from a few thousand to more than 300,000 in 2,000 settlements. Research has shown that members of MST communities enjoyed better health than other agricultural workers. The improved health of MST community members was attributed to a higher production of livestock, better nutrition (partly due to a greater diversity of produce), community support in case of need and direct involvement in community decisions. MST has acted as a catalyst for reform, not only agrarian reform, but also reform of health, with a direct impact on governmental decisions and an influence on public policies (EMCONET, 2007).

It is important that social movements are not too extreme in their views, and should be adaptable and willing to change their strategy to gain public and professional support. The Gay Liberation Front (see Box 2.2) is a movement that was too extreme, for the time, in its views and tactics and therefore had to create a more moderate organisation willing to engage with others that had differing points of view from its own.

Box 2.2   The Gay Liberation Front

The Gay Liberation Front (GLF) was a short-lived gay rights organisation initially founded in New York City in 1969 that spread to other cities with sizable gay and lesbian populations, especially on the West Coast, until its demise in the early

1970s. The organisation worked within the broader movement on gay rights but struggled to gain support because of its extreme views and internal conflicts. What distinguished the GLF from earlier organisations within the gay and lesbian communities was its rejection of integrationist approaches that sought civil rights for gay people within straight society and its call for active resistance to the entire heterosexist social order. Like the broader youth counterculture of the period, active resistance for GLF gays and lesbians meant being as expressive and shocking as possible. Earlier homophile groups argued that gays and lesbians were just like heterosexuals, except in their same-sex orientation. GLF members openly challenged the sexual binaries of homosexual and heterosexual as one of the many forms of oppression constraining everyone in American society. Membership in the GLF was based on gay pride and revolutionary commitment and in principle was open to all, regardless of gender, race, or any other social category. Yet, GLF activists tended to be predominantly young, white, male, and educated. As with other New Left organisations from this period, meetings were unstructured and democratic, with action by consensus. But, from the beginning, the GLF faced internal tension between gay men and lesbians, so much so that women began organising their own lesbian liberation groups. Conflicts also emerged between GLF members who wanted to organise all gays and lesbians into their own unique counterculture and those who wanted to join up with other revolutionary movements of the time. Still other controversies surfaced over the use of violence for winning gay rights. These conflicts forced a split in the GLF resulting in a new organisation, called the Gay Activists Alliance, that rejected the use of violence, advocated using the existing political structure to make pro-gay changes in society and focused entirely on gay-rights causes rather than building coalitions with other movements. By 1972, most GLF groups had fragmented and members drifted into other gay and lesbian movement organisations (Mirola, 2007a).

The genital integrity activists provide another example (see Box 2.3) of why an activist organisation should sometimes be prepared to be flexible and to change its agenda in view of public and professional opinion.

Box 2.3   The genital integrity activists

The genital integrity activists (**intactivists**) oppose genital modifications, including genital mutilation and sexual reassignment surgery and are committed to the recognition of the right to an intact body. They also oppose genital modifications that are medically harmful such as circumcision, whether male or female, and challenge the idea that circumcision is a healthy and beneficial procedure.

(Continued)

(Continued)

Intactivists disseminate information supporting their argument based on the outcomes of medical research. The International Coalition for Genital Integrity is a cooperation of some 30 civil society organisations, the majority of which are based in the USA. Campaigns of the coalition have not been very influential for two main reasons: first, while they have managed to base their opposition on the results of medical research, the view that circumcision is healthy and even required has strong support from the medical profession; second, the issue of genital modification, especially circumcision, is contentious given that it is practised by two religions: Islam and Judaism. Opposition to this by intactivists on the grounds that it is a violation of human rights, and an unhealthy practice does not therefore receive much public or professional support (Cakmak, 2007).

Health social movements

The growing awareness of health science that has become available through, for example, the internet, has led to people challenging health policy. This has been coupled by the negative publicity received about biomedical abuses, for example, experimentation with contraceptives, radiation and immunisation that has created a heightened level of distrust by the public. People have discovered that collectively they can apply significant pressure to influence policy that affects their health at both an individual and a collective level (Brown and Zavestoski, 2004). Health Social Movements (HSMs) ultimately challenge state, institutional and other forms of authority to give the public more of a voice in health policy and regulation. Health Social Movements are an important point of social interaction concerning the rights of people to access health services, personal experiences of illness, disease, disability and health inequality based on race, class, gender and sexuality. HSMs overlap in their purpose and tactics but can be categorised into three types (Brown et al., 2004: 685–686):

1. Health access movements that seek equitable access to health care services, for example, through national health care reforms and an extension of health insurance to non-insured sectors of the population.
2. Embodied health movements concern people who want to address personal experiences of disease, illness and disability through a challenge of the scientific evidence by medical recognition of their ideas or their own research. It can include people directly affected by a condition or those who feel they are an at risk group, for example, the HIV/AIDS movement.
3. Constituency-based health movements concern health inequalities when the evidence shows an oversight or disproportionate outcome, for example, the human rights movement.

The women's health movement in the 1970s and 1980s was a feminist-based medial approach that viewed the medical establishment as patriarchal, authoritarian, racist and demeaning to women. It focused on reproductive health issues and many women's groups started actions and clinics, run by women to help women for contraceptive and gynaecological services. Later the women's health movement became more independent and not directly connected to the women's rights or feminist movements (Baird et al., 2009). The environmental breast cancer movement in the USA was an example of the earlier efforts of women to gain more control over their reproductive health and was concerned with both equitable access to health care services and to addressing health inequalities with regard to women. The movement was formed by a spill-over from the women's movement, AIDS activism and the environmental movements. Maren Klawiter (2004) discusses the early experiences of women with breast cancer in the 1970s in the San Francisco Bay Area who endured isolation and power inequalities structured around the doctor-patient relationship. This HSM was created to identify with those at risk from or affected by breast cancer and provided many people with the intellectual and emotional support they needed to be able to move forward collectively to address a personal issue. Using the lessons that they had brought with them, they pressed for expanded clinical trials, compassionate access to new drugs and greater government funding. This HSM used tactics such as engaging in legal action, support to new research, creative media campaigns and influencing the policy process (Brown and Zavestoski, 2004). Twenty years later, a new breast cancer regime had emerged influenced by the efforts of the environmental breast cancer movement. Women had access to user-friendly cancer centres, patient education workshops, support groups, a choice of medical alternatives and a role as part of the health care team that delivered the cancer treatment. Essentially, breast cancer had become politicised and reframed as a feminist issue and an environmental disease.

International activist movements

The following is a summary of three key international activist movements: the Campaign for Nuclear Disarmament, environmentalism, and the animal rights movement. This is followed by the key lessons that can be drawn from the strategies that movements have used, what works and what does not work in activism.

The Campaign for Nuclear Disarmament

The Campaign for Nuclear Disarmament (CND) acts non-violently to rid the world of nuclear weapons and other weapons of mass destruction to create security for future generations. It opposes the development, manufacture, test-ing, deployment and use or threatened use by any country of these weapons. CND has a number of campaigns to address these issues including 'No to trident', 'Global abolition' and 'No to US missile defence' (Campaign for Nuclear Disarmament, 2012). In the 1950s, Europe was gripped by a very real fear of nuclear conflict and, building on the work of earlier anti-war movements, CND was launched. CND's advocacy of unilateral nuclear disarmament, the proposal that Britain should take the initiative and get rid of its own nuclear weapons, irrespective of the actions of others, caught the public imagination and from the outset all sections of society have been involved. There is always conflict within movements and in CND this was about whether to use illegal actions rather than more moderate yet still unconventional strategies such as civil disobedience, sit-ins and blockades. The principles and practices were eventually worked out so that when CND came to the fore again in the 1980s, non-violent, indirect strategies were the generally accepted form of action. For example, in September 1981, a mainly women's march from Cardiff arrived at Greenham Common US Air Force base in Berkshire, where the first Cruise missiles were to be stored. This soon became a permanent peace camp independent of CND, although many individual CND women members supported or joined the camp. The actions of CND now rely on a different sort of protest from the mass demonstrations of the past to address new issues such as nuclear production, transport and waste storage, radioactive leaks and the sale of nuclear explosives such as plutonium. The emphasis is now on the lobbying of MPs, on tracking and publicising road and rail shipments of nuclear materials as well as providing information to people and other interest groups (Byrne, 1988; Campaign for Nuclear Disarmament, 2012).

Environmentalism

Environmentalism is an ideology regarding concerns for environmental conservation and improvement of the health of the environment. In general terms, environmentalists advocate for the sustainable management of resources, and the protection of the environment through changes in public policy and individual behaviour. Environmentalist strategies influence the political process by lobbying, activism and education (Gibson, 2003) although photography and key publications have also been used to raise public awareness of environmental issues such as air pollution and petroleum spills. The early social movements that were formed, notably Greenpeace and Friends of the Earth, were intent on non-violent actions as a means of highlighting environmental injustices and raising issues for public debate. Greenpeace was founded in 1971 and is now an international non-governmental organisation known for its campaigns to fight against environmental degradation and to conserve the Earth's biodiversity (Greenpeace International, 2012).

To maintain its independence, Greenpeace does not accept donations from governments or corporations and relies on contributions from individual supporters, foundation grants and volunteerism. Radical pressure groups such as the Earth Liberation Front operate as covert cells and regularly use strategies such as economic sabotage and the destruction of property (Best and Nocella, 2006). Greenpeace has also received criticism because some of its members have been arrested for offences such as trespass, ship blockades, public demonstrations and, for example, tactics to prevent high seas whaling described in Box 2.4 below (Murguía, 2007a).

Box 2.4   Greenpeace and activist strategies

Greenpeace uses a strategy of combined tactics to address its key issues, for example, its approach on high seas whaling has employed a vessel, the *Steve Irwin*, to harass Japanese whaling boats in waters 300 miles north of Mawson Peninsula in Antarctica. When three anti-whaling activists were injured in a clash with Japanese whalers it made headline news (Shadbolt, 2012). Greenpeace and the Japanese government engaged in a media battle to convey their interpretation of events. At the same time, Greenpeace posted a video recording on what had happened on its website (Greenpeace International, 2012) and the same images also appeared on YouTube. The Greenpeace website urges people to send an email to Japan's Foreign Minister, providing easy access and a pre-written letter, regarding corrupt practices in Japanese whaling research. The website also provides information, fact sheets and images and satellites can be monitored that are tracking whales to expose the activities of Japanese research vessels.

Environmentalism has had to evolve to deal with new issues such as global warming, dumping waste onto disadvantaged communities, pollution and the exposure of organic life to toxins. The movement has become a more diverse scientific, social, and political movement but has also created specialist areas of concern such environmental justice. Environmental justice groups are especially active in highlighting the detrimental health affects of environmental pollution on socially disadvantaged groups in society (Bullard and Johnson, 2000). An example of the devastating affect that environmental pollution can have on poor communities is given in Box 2.5 below in regard to the Bhopal gas tragedy.

Box 2.5   The Bhopal gas tragedy

The Bhopal gas tragedy occurred between 2 and 3 December 1984 at the Union Carbide India Limited (UCIL) pesticide plant in India. A leak of methyl isocyanate gas and other chemicals resulted in the exposure of hundreds of thousands of people to toxic chemicals. The immediate death toll was 2,259 people and the government of Madhya Pradesh later confirmed a total of 3,787 deaths related to the gas release. Other estimates are much higher and a government affidavit in 2006 stated the leak caused 558,125 injuries including 38,478 partial and approximately 3,900 severely and permanently disabling injuries. UCIL was the Indian subsidiary of Union Carbide Corporation (UCC) in the USA. In June 2010, seven ex-employees, including the former UCIL chairman, were convicted in Bhopal of causing death by negligence and

(Continued)

(Continued)

sentenced to two years' imprisonment, the maximum punishment allowed by law. A group of Bhopal activists in America held a demonstration outside the Indian Embassy, demanding that the Indian Prime Minister provide justice to the Bhopal gas tragedy victims and extradite the then Union Carbide chief to India. They held demonstrations in front of the Gandhi statue and submitted a petition to the Prime Minister of India through the Embassy in the United States. The activists called their movement the International Campaign for Justice in Bhopal and demanded a cleaning up of the site in Bhopal and greater compensation to the victims of the tragedy (Oneindia, 2010).

A sub-set of environment justice groups are **community-based ecological resistance movements** that emerge within struggles against environmental degradation. These are devoted to the protection of community life from environmentally harmful activities and to mobilise people in resistance to the issue. The awareness that the community lives with and within the environment is the key factor in the political mobilisation of community members. Community-based ecological resistance movements differ from other types of environmental movements, such as single-issue local movements, nature conservationist movements, and mainstream environmental movements, because they specifically aim to protect community-environment interactions in a particular locality. The environment is not conceived as raw materials but is based on its significance for the spiritual, cultural, social, and economic life of its communities. It is a strategy for self-defence and prompts a spontaneous direct resistance movement aimed at protecting the community's well-being.

Strategies that have been employed by community-based ecological resistance movements have relied on community activism, local leadership, and resource mobilisation and have ranged from militant and sometimes illegal, such as road blockades and **crop trashing** (see Box 2.6), to non-violent, peaceful actions such as press conferences, petitions, lobbying and demonstrations (Plows, 2007).

Box 2.6   Crop trashing

Crop trashing developed as part of a tactical repertoire in the UK in the late 1990s, with the government policy decision to grow field-scale trials for genetically modified (GM) crops. Crop squats were protest camps in fields that were to be planted with a GM crop. Many overt crop trashes happened when rallies at the GM field sites turned into mass trespasses where the participants damaged the crops. A favoured tactic was covert trashing, whereby unknown and probably multiple groups of activists, thought to be operating in groups, were responsible for the sudden destruction of a large number of field trial sites (Plows, 2007).

Though it is often a long and expensive strategy, activists also use the tactic of legal actions by filing administrative appeals and lawsuits. Taking legal action usually helps exert the pressure of the law on administrative authorities or corporations responsible for activities harmful to the environment. The Bergama movement in Turkey is an interesting example in this respect. The villagers' resistance was against an 'open pit' gold mining investment by a multinational corporation in the small town of Bergama. Heavily engaged in agriculture, they saw the mine as a threat to community life, the environment, and future generations. The early mobilisations took the form of meetings, press conferences, and petitions to declare their opposition. The movement started when community members blocked the main road connecting two big cities to protest at the felling of thousands of olive trees for the 'open pit' operation. As the corporation (backed by the Turkish government) insisted on putting the mine into operation, the community persisted with the demand for the cessation of its activities by employing confrontational tactics not only in their region but also around the country. They also took legal action against the government authorities that issued mining permits to allow the corporation to commence gold extraction. Despite the court decisions emphasising the right to healthy living and a healthy environment, the mining activity continued while the villagers' struggle went on in the courts and on the streets. Alliances with professional organisations, environmentalist groups, trade unions, and human rights activists helped the movement to make the local conflict a national issue. The struggle politicised the community as almost all members with no previous experience in any political activism except voting became committed to defend the cause (Coban and Yetis, 2007).

The animal rights movement

The animal liberation movement, sometimes called the animal rights movement, animal personhood, or animal-advocacy movement, is a social movement which seeks an end to the moral and legal distinction between humans and animals. The movement aims to include animals in society by putting their basic interests on an equal footing with the basic interests of human beings, for example, not being made to suffer pain on behalf of humans or animals. The movement includes many sub-groups covering issues such as animal welfare (RSPCA and Animal Aid) that have a charitable status and use conventional approaches. The animal liberation movement is regarded as having been founded in the UK in the early 1970s and was later supported by a wide variety of academics and professionals, including lawyers, physicians, psychologists, veterinarians, and former vivisectionists in Europe and North America (Encyclopædia Britannica, 2007). As animal liberationists became increasingly influenced by activism, the term '**veganarchists**' was developed as a philosophy of veganism and activism. This encompasses viewing the state as unnecessary and harmful to animals whilst observing a vegan diet. The animal rights movement has received public and professional support for its cause, for example in the USA support is given by the Humane Society of the USA (animal protection) and the Physicians' Committee for Responsible Medicine (animal rights). The movement has been successful, for example, in Germany which guaranteed rights to animals in a 2002 amendment to its constitution, becoming the first EU member to do so. Another success of the animal liberation movement has been the granting of basic rights to five great ape species in New Zealand in 1999. Their use is now forbidden in research, testing or teaching. Most animal rights groups reject violence against persons, intimidation, threats, and the destruction of property. Instead they concentrate on education, research and media campaigns (Brian, 1997). However, the Animal Rights Movement has become associated with a variety of activist methods, some quite extreme, because of the actions of individuals and small independent groups. On 1 March 2007, for example, Belgian and Dutch police carried out 32 separate police raids, involving 700 police officers, the largest ever effort at suppressing the animal rights movement in Europe (UK Animal Rights, 2011). Other activist groups operate in covert cells consisting of small numbers of trusted friends, or of individuals acting alone, using names like the Animal Liberation Front (ALF). These cells engage in direct action, for example, by carrying out raids to release animals from laboratories or by boycotting and targeting anyone or any business associated with animal testing laboratories. Arson and vandalism have been linked to animal liberation groups carrying out 'open rescues' in which liberationists enter businesses to remove animals without trying to hide their identities, risking arrest. For example, Barry Horne was an animal liberation activist who died in a UK prison hospital on 5 November 2001 following a third hunger strike. He had been sentenced to 18 years in prison for criminal damage and arson attacks mainly against companies involved in vivisection. In prison, he went on hunger strike several times in protest against government support for the vivisection industry and his actions helped to generate worldwide publicity (Francione, 1996; Newkirk, 2000; UK Animal Rights, 2011).

Counter tactics by commercial and corporate interests

Many large commercial and corporate lobbies have far more influence than ordinary citizens, pressure groups or social movements. Companies are of course part of civil society and contribute in many positive ways but they can also put their interests ahead of the public interest and find political allies in trying to marginalise or counter the tactics used by activist groups that are against their agenda. Corporations use a range of public relations tactics designed to influence decision makers, researchers, public opinion and policy analysis (Hager, 2009). There are sophisticated public relations, market research and lobbying companies specialising in these types of counter-activist tactics in support of, and often only within the financial reach of, corporations.

Corporations fund paid experts to speak to the media. A classic example of this is the paid voices from the finance sector (bank economists, merchant bank spokespeople etc.) who are regularly treated as independent commentators on economic issues in the media but who are paid to promote policies that favour their employers. Corporate media campaigns employ sophisticated media management companies to help define and shape issues using well-funded advertising campaigns. A major part of this type of public relations work is attacking opponents and trying to stop them having a 'voice', such as persistently targeting public health researchers working on a specific issue in a way that intimidates them and distracts them from their work. Meanwhile, these companies cultivate and support favourable researchers by providing helpful funding, travel opportunities and conferences. Corporations also routinely seek community or professional groups as 'third parties' to confirm and to give credibility to their messages publicly. When groups cannot be won over, false scientific and community groups have become an alternative 'tool'. These are the groups that quickly emerge to support large developments or to defend unpopular corporations such as smokers' rights groups. Frequently the lobby groups present themselves publicly as independent and/or science-based, for example, pharmaceutical companies will establish consumer and patient groups in pursuit of their own interests or engage with existing groups in the debate on policy proposals to add legitimacy to their activities (Allsop et al., 2004). The well-resourced interest groups can hire lawyers to put pressure on planned or existing government policies by threatening judicial review and other time-consuming legal challenges. Another major tool of influence is election donations. In New Zealand for example, the alcohol and tobacco industry has been funding political parties and gaining influence for the last century (Hager, 2009).

There are also corporate gifts where politicians and other targeted people of influence are given free tickets to important sporting events, concerts and cultural events provided by industry interests. Some industries are more aggressive than others. Generally the more controversial they are, the more they have to hide or the more negative the externalities of their business are, the more considerable resources are invested in these tactics. Some corporations, such as from the tobacco industry, use sponsorship for low-cost marketing such as paying trivial sums for school road-crossing jackets with logos displayed on them, advertising, community events or providing grants for community development activities.

Corporate social responsibility (CSR) also called corporate conscience, corporate citizenship, social performance, or responsible business is a form of self-regulation integrated into a business plan or model. CSR policy functions as a built-in mechanism whereby a business monitors and ensures its active compliance with the spirit of the law, ethical standards and international best practices. The goal of CSR is to embrace responsibility for the company's actions and encourage a positive impact through its activities. Promoting 'corporate social responsibility' reports has become one of the growth areas in the corporate public relations industry. Companies have formed specialist CSR practice groups with the role of embracing accountability and transparency as a means to build corporate credibility and reputation. For example, manufacturing companies that have been criticised for employing child labour, thus potentially damaging their 'corporate image', have devoted much greater attention to developing, overseeing and reporting on new labour standards of suppliers and their sub-contractors as part of a counter campaign (see Box 2.7).

Box 2.7   Child labour and counter campaigning

Child labour refers to the employment of children at regular and sustained work. This practice is considered exploitative by many international organisations and is illegal in many countries. Child labour can be detrimental to the early development of children and has an effect on their health for their entire life. Child labour laws are the legal guidelines in place to prevent or regulate the employment of children. However, child labour is still common, in, for example, factory work, mining, prostitution, agriculture and in the informal sector such as selling items on the street or begging, in many developing countries. Stop Firestone (Stop Firestone, 2012) is a campaign of the Stop Firestone Coalition, a group made up of both US- and Liberia-based organisations. One key focus has been the Firestone Tire and Rubber Company's operation in Liberia including a rubber plantation in which children were reported to have been made to work excessively long hours to fulfil a high production quota. The Firestone Tire and Rubber Company denied these claims and started a concerted counter campaign stating that it has helped families and children through education and has applied better employment standards. However, the International Labour Rights Fund filed a lawsuit against the company in 2005 on behalf of current child labourers and their parents who had also worked on the plantation as children. In 2007, Firestone's motion to dismiss the case was denied and the lawsuit was allowed to proceed (Knudsen, 2007).

Corporations can, for example, use one of four main counter strategies: deflect, defer, dismiss or defeat. Opposing stakeholders with power but no passion should be 'deflected' to avoid their involvement in the situation. People with passion but no power, on the other hand, can be 'defeated', for example through reaching a compromise. And people with neither passion nor power are 'dismissed'. Countering activist actions by organisations that have both high passion and high power may require the company to 'defer' to their demands. Even if companies are reluctant, their best strategy is to engage with activists, to sell an idea and to try and divide and conquer. Once engaged, activists often don't notice, or turn a blind eye to, the dual corporate strategy of collaborating with activists while also lobbying behind the scenes to weaken existing regulations or undermine other campaigns. The benefits of the collaboration with corporations can include better opportunities for funding. The cost of long-term collaboration is a greater identification with corporations' policy agendas rather than advocating greater social justice (Burton, 2007).

What works and what does not in activism

There are a number of lessons that can be drawn from the international experiences of activism of what works and what does not work including the strategies used by social movements, pressure groups and community-based organisations. These key lessons are as follows:

1. Frame the strategy and tactics around a single, simple issue (rather than multiple, complex problems).
2. Use simple messaging with clear policy solutions delivered through, for example, media advocacy to raise awareness about your cause.
3. Frame the issue to gain supportive public and professional opinion for your cause. Professional and public opposition to your cause will greatly reduce your chances of success.
4. Activists have to be patient for, or strive to create, the particular circumstances that are most likely to produce a supportive political environment.
5. Activism backed by legal action has been one of the most effective means of achieving policy change.
6. Using an aggressive marketing approach in health advocacy can have an influence on policy.
7. Networking is an important means to bring people together to share ideas either through a physical meeting or through social network internet sites.
8. Peaceful civil protests and demonstrations help to gain media attention and reframe the health debate and are more effective if part of a broader strategy, for example, using media advocacy and legal action.
9. Using the mass media can help to shift public opinion if it is also followed up with a professional and public debate about the key issues, over a prolonged period of time.
10. Sophisticated advertising campaigns do require a large budget and are therefore an expensive strategy to gain public and professional support.
11. Unconventional actions such as hacking into another computer ('**Hacktivism**') to obtain information or damage to private property can result in negative public opinions or prosecutions.
12. Activist organisations must be prepared to be moderate, adaptable and willing to change their strategy, for example, the Gay Liberation Front were too extreme, for the time, in their views and tactics and had to shift their position to be willing to engage with mainstream political processes.
13. The ability of the organisation to create an alliance or **partnership** with influential others who can act as 'champions' for their cause can be an effective strategy.
14. Activist organisations must be prepared to evolve to take advantage of the interconnection of electronic-based networks and **information and communication technologies** for effective activist strategies.

The strength of activist organisations lies less in numbers and more in assets such as strong leadership, evidence-backed positions, good media relations, a network of strategic alliances with other groups, the ability to use multiple strategies, organisational structures and sufficient, independent financial resources. An activist organisation must eventually become self-sustaining, or it fades away. Organisations that hold a charitable status are often dependent on government funding and are reluctant to engage in activist tactics because this can attract negative publicity and result in a reduced source of income. Receiving funding in this way compromises the strength of their tactics and on their ability to 'attack' government. Some organisations, for example, Greenpeace, do not accept government funding so as to maintain their independence.

The policy analysis of activist organisations shows that the most effective strategies use a combination of conventional and unconventional tactics. In particular, legal action, media advocacy and the mass media combined with mass protests or media stunts can have a dramatic effect in changing public opinion. In South Africa, for example, a case by-passing the courts and going to the country's Competition Commission, successfully argued that the high prices for anti-Retro viral drugs levied by two big drug companies violated regulations against excessive pricing and South Africa's guarantee of the 'right to life' (Labonté and Schrecker, 2007). Advocacy has more impact if it can focus on immediate issues that are already known to the public. The campaign should limit itself to one or two consistent and easily memorised key messages supported by a large movement of people to voice their concern and to share the message with others (Galer-Unti, 2009).

Some organisations have charitable status, a type of not-for-profit organisation. The legal definition of a charitable organisation varies according to the country in which it operates as do the charitable purposes such as faith organisations, the aged, homeless and addressing the special needs of vulnerable persons. To publicly raise funds, charities in most countries are required to register under the state jurisdiction within which they intend to operate (Charity Commission, 2012; Fitzroy Legal Service Inc, 2012). Charities are dependent on private donations and government funding and are therefore reluctant to engage in activism that may attract negative publicity, for example, unconventional tactics such as media stunts. Charities usually do not consider themselves to be 'activists' and rely on tactics such as advocacy, education, lobbying and networking. The status as a charity can create a dependence on funding sources including the government and this means that the organisation has to be cautious about attracting negative publicity. There is, however, an advantage of a strategy that allows unconventional tactics by individuals who do not associate themselves with the movement itself but do associate themselves with the movement's cause. Bad publicity because of radical tactics is viewed by the media as the responsibility of the individual and not the movement. However, any gain, for example, from positive publicity may also be received by the movement that supports the cause.

In a rapidly changing world, activist tactics are evolving to take advantage of information and communication technology (ICT), such as the World Wide Web, the internet, Twitter, Facebook and the Short Message Service. This is helping activist organisations to communicate better, to organise, to mobilise, to lever and to raise resources for their respective causes. There is also an increasingly important role for ICT in social networking for quickly bringing people together and for re-framing the debate around activist issues. The use of ICT is rapidly changing the way in which people are able to mobilise themselves for mass advocacy through the use of tactics that can target individuals and organisations requiring a minimum of resources, for example, 'virtual sit-ins' and e-petitions.

Unconventional actions such as civil disobedience with the intention to carry out physical damage on property or persons have led to prosecutions. Placing oneself in a position of manufactured vulnerability to prevent action such as a 'lock-on' is also a risky tactic and can result in negative public opinion. This type of negative publicity can deter people from joining or donating to an activist organisation (Brashers et al., 2002). However, some activists seem to be willing to take these risks in an attempt to raise public awareness (positively or negatively) about their cause. There is a dual strategy used by some activist movements: one is moderate and conventional whilst the other is radical and uses extreme tactics that in practice can result in dynamic outcomes. Social movements, pressure and advocacy groups can choose from a wide range of tactics to influence the opinions and actions of others including policymakers and the general public. What defines an activist organisation or group is whether or not it is willing to use tactics that go beyond what is considered to be conventional. Next, in Chapter 3 I discuss the controversial role of health practitioners, and the organisations and institutions that employ them, in health activism.

3

Activism and the health practitioner

Health programming

Health programming aims to promote health, prevent disease, treat illnesses, prolong valued life, care for the infirm and to provide health services. Traditionally, such goals have been used to curb the spread of infectious diseases and to protect the well-being of the general population whilst others see a much greater role in regulation and reducing inequalities in health (Baggott, 2000). The range of goals also means that it covers a number of preventive and promotion specialist areas including environmental health, nursing, public health and health promotion and not surprisingly has a wide range of competing perspectives, priorities and services. Health programmes are most commonly implemented as activities managed and monitored by a practitioner and/or an agency such as state departments or government-funded agencies, trusts, foundations and non-governmental organisations. The programme typically includes a period of identification, design, appraisal, approval, implementation and evaluation. It is summarised as aims and objectives, identifying in advance suitable indicators of progress and the prior assessment of risks and assumptions. Health practitioners are also employed to deliver the information, resources and services that form the programme design. In practice, health programmes still belong primarily to people employed in the health sector, in the sense that it provides these workers with some conceptual models, professional legitimacy and resources. These people may be titled 'health promoters' or 'health educators' while many more who look to the idea of health occupy jobs such as environmental health officers, nurses and doctors. In this book, I refer to all these people as the 'practitioner(s)'. It is the health practitioner or their agency that usually also chooses the selection of 'targeted groups' and the methods to be used to reach them in top-down programmes. Similarly, the initiation of the programme, the issues to be addressed and the enthusiasm for its direction are often led by the practitioner. Health programming entails a power relationship between different stakeholders, primarily between the practitioner, and their agencies, often representing the state, and their clients. The clients are the people, groups and communities who are the recipients of the information, resources and services being delivered to promote health. The practitioners in a programme are often in a position of relative power to the people who benefit from the programme, for example, they usually have control of allocating limited resources, selecting who is to receive training, education and advisory services.

Practitioners that are employed through institutional settings consist of a number of distinctive positions of control with specialist duties that are usually formally defined. The officials who hold these positions of power are recruited according to specific rules and their employment is usually based on a system of salaries. Power is hierarchically top-down and the official is expected to act in accordance with, and without challenging, the instructions descending from their superiors (Turner and Samson, 1995). An example of a highly institutional and hierarchical health organisation is a hospital or a government department. Positioning oneself within the hierarchy of an institutional setting provides a practitioner legitimacy and status. This is achieved not necessarily because that person has particular expertise but because the institutionalisation of the position creates the idea that she/he is an expert. Within institutional settings, practitioners can be attributed more occupational autonomy over the process by which a particular service is delivered, for example, individual nurses who did not have to always seek approval for every action were found to act more autonomously than on a closely managed ward (Kendall, 1998). If it is true that health is an institutionalised activity, carried out by or within governmental organisations or government funded agencies, it is also true that many of these organisations remain loyal to traditional ways of thinking and acting, ways which inhibit the effective inclusion of empowering approaches. Various studies of both government and non-government organisations have found that the concept of empowerment used in policy and in practice is often quite different (Grace, 1991). Despite the intent to 'empower' communities, the organisations and their staff tended to retain control over programming rather than to relinquish power to others. The agencies operated within a contradiction between discourse and practice. Many practitioners continued to exert power-over the beneficiaries through top-down programming whilst at the same time using emancipatory discourse (Laverack, 1999).

Before practitioners can empower others, they must first be themselves empowered and understand the sources of their own power. To build a more empowering practice, health programmes must redress the constraints placed on the profession by its institutional nature and by the institutional culture that does not necessarily share an ideology of empowerment. This has been argued in the context of a nursing profession that cannot be empowered unless individual nurses themselves are empowered and can be extended to an institutional work setting such as a hospital, a community of both patients and staff. Both must be empowered and this includes feeling valued and having the resources, skills and knowledge to empower others (Kendall, 1998). Nurses work to enable patients to take more control in decision making over their health, promoting patient independence, information exchange and being aware of their needs. In practice, this translates into acts of care such as making sure patients have their call bell within reach, respecting their choices, providing information about future care options and working quietly at night to allow patients to sleep (Faulkner, 2001). An empowerment approach gives even more credibility to what the individual has to offer in patient centred care and goes beyond self-care to what the individual can offer to improve the system. An individualistic approach focuses on supporting people to make informed choices, relationship building, self-management and partnerships. The broader empowerment of patients enables them to have an influence on the health system through networking and engagement with patient advocacy and pressure groups. The purpose is therefore collective action, as well as individual self-care.

Governments and the bureaucracies that they create, at least in democratic countries, are not monolithic entities. Not only are there often contradictions between the policies and actions of different government agencies but different practitioners with differing ideas often exist and work together. Practitioners working in large institutional settings can find their autonomy being undermined by the hierarchical structure of rules and lines of control, or else their power base is encroached upon by para-practitioner groups. These circumstances actually present opportunities for an empowering practice to develop within even the largest, most rigid bureaucracies. To take advantage of these opportunities, the practitioner must understand better how to use the structures and procedures of their agencies to facilitate working at the interface with the community. Examples include the involvement of community representatives on advisory committees or the provision of grants based on expressed community needs rather than on programme goals. It is precisely this type of an issue that must be addressed if practitioners are to engage an empowering approach in their daily work. Practitioners must also make the decision to gain the necessary skills and knowledge, if they are committed to an approach that will empower others in health programmes.

The role of the health practitioner

The role of the health practitioner has traditionally been one of enforcer, of educationalist or as an enabler of empowerment. In this book I discuss a fourth role, that of health activist or at least one of supporting others to undertake health activism.

The public image of the practitioner's role as an enforcer of health legislation, for example, has been supported by the work of government employees such as environmental health departments that are concerned with inspection, licensing, complaint investigations and legal proceedings. An enforcement of the wide range of public health protection and food safety legislation has been seen to be necessary to maintain a healthy and safe environment in the home, at work and during recreation. The role of the health enforcer has helped to establish the image of some practitioners having power-over their clients through the use of legislation and has led to terms such as 'sanitary policemen'.

The second role of the practitioner has been concerned with education, training and specialist services, for example, that of a nurse providing advice to a group of young mothers or giving treatment to their patients. This role has helped to broaden the image of the practitioner holding 'expert' power and access to technical resources, skills and knowledge. Expert power stems from others attributing superior knowledge and ability to the health practitioner; for example, the term 'doctor knows best' illustrates the expert relationship between patient and doctor. This creates a social role relationship between the practitioner and their client, a structural relationship that grants the practitioner the right to prescribe certain behaviours which the other person accepts as an obligation to comply with.

The third role of the practitioner, one that has developed more recently and that is complementary to their roles as enforcers, educators and specialists, is how their day-to-day work can be empowering for others. At the heart of this role is the ability of the practitioner to transform their own power-over (access to information, resources and expertise) to a power-with relationship in which their clients are helped to gain more power. The outcome is that individuals, groups and communities are helped to gain greater control over decision making and access to resources in regard to their health. The qualities of an empowering relationship include a non-coercive dialogue in the identification of problems and actions to resolve problems through autonomous choice. Informed and autonomous choice is core to empowerment approaches since it must be the individual, group or community who are active in changing their own circumstances. Autonomy refers to the capacity to be self-governing, to making the decisions that will influence one's life and health. It is linked to what it is to be a person, to be able to choose freely and to be able to formulate how one wants to live one's life. It is also related to having the freedom and opportunities in our lives to be able to make the right choices for ourselves (Kant, 2004). The key attributes of the practitioner in an empowering role are as an enabler, helper, counsellor and guide to support others to facilitate change in their lives through their own actions.

Not all practitioners can apply the fourth role as an activist to their everyday work. For example, those involved in enforcement, licensing and legal proceedings will have fewer opportunities than those working in an advisory, counselling or community development role. This is because enforcement uses a power-over approach to maintain authority in contrast to an advisory and educational role that can use a power-with approach to build the power-from-within of other people. An empowering practitioner relationship involves the ability to be a good communicator, a good listener, helping people to become more critically aware and linking individuals to groups that share their needs and interests. Activism takes the empowerment role even further to a point where the practitioner works with others to enable them to gain more control using unconventional tactics. This role is explicitly driven by goals for political change manifest as new or favourable changes to policy and legislation. Practitioners also have the right and therefore an option of exercising their own voices as citizens, for example, through their participation in social movements. In the same way, practitioners can act as professional advocate groups to support the actions of others who they believe suffer from a health inequality. They can endorse the concerns of these less powerful groups by using their 'expert power' to legitimise their concerns. For example, the support of the medical profession to the advocacy group Action on Smoking and Health (ASH) has given credibility to this cause and in some European countries has contributed to a nationwide ban in public places because of the associated health risks of passive smoking. Likewise, the British Medical Association has given its support to the political lobby for the stricter legal regulation of boxing (Brayne et al., 1998) based on health grounds.

Philosophical considerations

Per-Anders Tengland (2007), a health philosopher, believes that the logic for using an empowering approach is justified because it is well founded and ethically and morally sound to do so. Tengland concludes from a conceptual analysis of collective empowerment that as a means or as a process it has applicability for creating freedom and opportunity to improve health. However, he questions if most practitioners have the knowledge and skills that are required to undertake an empowering approach. Practitioners often work with people from different cultural backgrounds and need to have a shared understanding if they are to use empowering approaches in their everyday work. This would include a better understanding of themselves, their beliefs and values and to put this into a framework of the relevant social and cultural perceptions.

The 'non-zero-sum' form of power conveniently shifts the focus away from awkward ethical and political issues concerning the underlying health determinants rooted in poverty, powerlessness and inequality (Labonté and Laverack, 2008). This form of power is 'win/win', based on the idea that if any one person or group gains, everyone else gains also. Knowledge, trust, caring and in particular, participation in social relationships, are examples of non-zero-sum power. Participation can help to promote involvement in health programmes, although it is generally agreed that participation alone does not lead to action or empowerment, does not lead to improved health outcomes and does not lead to improved health care (Rifkin, 2011). Participation offers a form of involvement without committing either the outside agency or the community to take further action. Perhaps unsurprisingly then, public health gravitates towards the non-zero-sum formulation by placing an emphasis on participation and responsibility to others, in which all people can benefit. Power is no longer seen as a finite commodity, such as wealth, or as the comparative status and authority that this might confer. Non-zero-sum power takes the form of respect, generosity, service to others, a free flow of information and a commitment to the ethics of caring and justice. The philosophical issue here is that practitioners continue to use terms such as participation without any real commitment to help communities to gain more power and their role then becomes mere rhetoric, paying 'lip-service' to empowerment.

Language exerts considerable force in our world constructions and this applies to our professional as well as our social worlds (Seidman and Wagner, 1992). In practice, the advantage is often held by the one with the power-over, usually the practitioner, and the language that they choose to use can either strengthen or weaken the professional relationship. Technical terms are a part of the everyday language of practitioners, for example, medical diagnostic vocabulary, and have evolved as knowledge and skills develop within a profession's subculture (other subcultures include ethnic groups, social class, sexuality). However, the use of specialist language is often confusing to both lay people and to practitioners who are not part of the professional subculture. This can contribute to their sense of powerlessness by showing a lack of access to knowledge and the 'expert' power of the other person using the language. The use of terms such as 'high risk' and 'target group' imply passivity and locate the problem within the group rather than in the relationship to the broader health determinants. Whilst it may sometimes be necessary to use specific technical terms it is more empowering when using language and terminology that is understood by the receivers. This reduces any confusion, alienation or mystification on behalf of the receiver by the communicator. The philosophical issue here is that the practitioner should be aware that no discourse is value-free. It is important to understand the influence of their language and to be sensitive to the position and perceptions of others. Such awareness is termed a 'reflexive practice' in which practitioners are critical about the way they use their knowledge and power to have influence over others. Scrambler (1987) provides an example of a consultation between a health practitioner and a pregnant woman. The practitioner began the discussion using 'lay' terms to describe the complications associated with her condition but quickly switched to a technical-rational language when her advice was challenged by the pregnant woman. The woman was then coerced into complying with the practitioner because she suddenly felt uncertain and lacking in knowledge. The pregnant woman had been disempowered by the practitioner who said that she was unaware of the switch to a technical, power-over use of language.

Ethical considerations

There is a good deal of discussion regarding the application of ethics to public health including a lively critical disassembling of definitions and models that suffused the 1980s and 1990s. David Seedhouse (1997), a health philosopher, suggests four simple points for an ethical approach that combine a blend of liberalism (provision of core resources but not a guarantee of full equality), utilitarianism (improve these core conditions for all rather than for particular 'groups') and egalitarianism (make this improvement a social priority for all):

1. a core respect for the autonomy of individuals;
2. a focus on central conditions in people's lives that support such autonomy;
3. prevention of disease, illness, injury and disability as legitimate health 'targets'; and
4. the prevention of obstacles in achieving the three points above.

In addition to these points, there are a number of key ethical questions in regard to the health practitioner, the health programme and the targeted beneficiaries of the programme.

Who, at the expense of others, should get priority for programme support and assistance?

David Zakus and Catherine Lysack (1998), two Canadian health researchers, argue that in practice we work from a zero-sum construction of power, increasing 'unhealthy' competition between people and groups and decreasing 'healthy' community cohesion. They suggest that 'community empowerment' is a contradiction in terms because by empowering some at the expense of others (zero-sum-power), we are actually breaking down the social ties that hold a community together.

Zero-sum power exists when one can only possess x amount of power to the extent that someone else has the absence of an equivalent amount. It is therefore a 'win/lose' situation. My power-over you, plus your absence of that power, equals zero (thus the term, 'zero-sum'). I win and you lose. For you to gain power, you must seize it from me. If you can, you win and I lose. By their very nature, communities consist of competing heterogeneous individuals and groups and public health, with limited resources, cannot avoid helping some whilst not others. The ethical issue here is which communities and groups, at the expense of others, should get priority to assist them to gain more control over resources or decision making that influence their lives and health. For example, if a local activist group successfully opposes the plans to site a toxic waste dump next to their community which is then shifted to another site where the community does not have the capacity to organise itself to oppose the relocation, what has been the gain in community empowerment (Baum, 2007)? In this case, the gain is localised because one 'community of interest' avoids the development of the waste dump, whilst another local community loses. Broader civil society, of which both communities are a part, has no gain in empowerment.

The priority of who receives access to the limited resources and assistance is often based upon which communities have the greatest need, the greatest inequalities in health and have the least socio-economic opportunities. The programming issue then becomes how to determine which communities to help relative to others in society. There are a number of indices that have been developed to assess poverty and social inequality for the prioritisation and distribution of resources and technical assistance. The Human Poverty Index, for example, developed by the UN provides an indication of the standard of living in a country, whereas for highly developed countries, the UN considers that it can better reflect the extent of deprivation using a comparison with the Human Development Index (UNDP, 2011).

What if the group in question is involved in unpalatable activities?

The issue of who to help can be confounded if the group in question is involved in illegal or unpalatable activities such as drug use or commercial sex or if the agenda set by the group does not match that of the implementing agency. For example, if parents request baby massage as part of a child health programme, the practitioner may feel that this does not enhance child health. The use of programme funds for this purpose, based on the evidence of what works, is ill advised (Braunack-Mayer and Louise, 2008) and might be more efficiently spent on promoting breastfeeding practices. In this case, funding baby massage is not a harmful practice, but it is an opportunity cost lost by the use of funds for an activity that is not actively beneficial. However, practitioners are employed to engage in programmes designed to improve or maintain the health of individuals, groups and communities. Practitioner groups within public health are expected to display a specialisation of knowledge, technical competence and social responsibility. Their level of practitionerism is attained through education, specialised training, testing of competence by formal examinations, the membership of a professional organisation and the inclusion of codes of practice (Turner and Samson, 1995). Practitioners are employed to deliver services and are not expected to be opinionated in regard to others, even though they may not agree on their activities. The ethical issue here is whether or not health practitioners should be allowed to choose with whom they work, whether they can apply their personal judgment and whether they should be excluded from working with others based on their own religious, moral or philosophical preferences.

Do people really want to be, or can they become, empowered?

One of the tensions that practitioners face is whether people actually want to be empowered. It is the practitioner, or their agency, that usually selects the programme beneficiaries and the methods to be used to help to empower them. The initiation of the empowerment process and the enthusiasm for its direction is often led by the practitioner. This is contradictory to an empowering approach in which the issue to be addressed and the means of reaching an empowered solution should be the responsibility of the beneficiaries of the programme, based on their own needs.

Some people may simply not want to become empowered. People, especially if they have lived in oppressive or powerless circumstances, may feel that they do not have the right or do not possess the motivation to empower themselves. Kieffer (1984: 16) provides an example of the experience of Sharon, a Native American living in Harlem: 'It would never have occurred to me to have expressed an opinion on anything ... It was inconceivable that my opinion had any value ... that's lower than powerlessness ... You don't even know the word "power" exists'. This internalisation of 'badness' leads to what is described as false consciousness, 'failing to utilize the power that one has and failing to acquire powers that one can acquire' (Morriss, 1987: 94). Learned helplessness is a similar psychological construct that emerged from Martin Seligman's animal research in the 1960s (Seligman and Maier, 1967). Dogs were subjected to inescapable electric shocks. When the barrier preventing their escape from these shocks was removed, the dogs continued to withstand them anyway and did not seek escape. Even if they accidentally avoided the shocks, they did not internalise this learning and continued to endure subsequent shocks. They had resigned themselves to their fate; they had 'learned helplessness'. The dogs, however, did 're-learn' how to escape after repeated 'teachings' by the researchers, in which the dogs were pushed, pulled or prodded away from the area being shocked. Martin Seligman has now coined another term, 'learned optimism', to encompass the dynamic of learning how to develop positive self-images (Seligman, 1990). Michael Lerner (1986), a political scientist and psychotherapist, argues that a similar phenomenon occurs with persons living in risk conditions. He named this process 'surplus powerlessness', a surplus created by, but distinct from, external or objective conditions of powerlessness. Individuals internalise powerlessness and this creates a potent psychological barrier to empowering action or other activities that meet their real needs. They accept aspects of their world that are self-destructive to their own well-being, thinking that these are unalterable features of what they take to be 'reality' (Lerner, 1986).

Do people have a right not to become empowered? What must be remembered is that power cannot be given but people must gain or seize it for themselves. The right to be empowered rests with the individual or group and the role of the practitioner is to facilitate and enable others to take greater responsibility and control over their lives. Some people may not want the responsibility of making decisions or fear the regret of making a misjudgement and therefore 'delegate' this authority to another person in whom they have trust. The example in Box 3.1 below illustrates this issue.

Box 3.1   The Early Intervention Programs

The Early Intervention Programs in Massachusetts, USA served infants and toddlers with developmental disabilities. Much of the practitioners' efforts working with children and parents were spent transmitting and reinforcing clinical knowledge, so that parents could work with their children and become empowered to advocate for others with special needs. However, parents with very young children (under the age of three), needed time to understand their children's conditions and the implications for their children and family, before taking action. If an advocacy expectation of the parents of children with disabilities is created it may be that many parents cannot or do not want to fulfil this role. This advocacy expectation puts the burden of change on parents, who do not control the distribution of power, nor the institutional practices that rectify it (Leiter, 2004). They then have the right to delegate the advocacy responsibility to another person or organisation to act on their behalf.

Other individuals, for example, the very young, the very old or people with an addiction, may not have the ability to organise and mobilise themselves towards collective empowerment. A key issue, for example, when working with children is at what age they begin to understand the social world in a concrete and abstract way such that they can fully engage with the concept of empowerment and the underlying, often political, causes of their powerlessness. An approach to childhood based on rights, or the participation agenda, sees children as social actors who act on the world around them. Practitioners can then engage with children about their worlds and involve them in decision making. Although there is not a definitive 'youngest' age at which children can be engaged to empower themselves collectively, my own inquiries into this issue have led to a guide of 14 years, give or take a year, depending on the individual. Empowerment interventions have been successfully used with adolescents (Wallerstein and Sanchez-Merki, 1994) but the successful engagement of children under the age of 14 years in empowerment approaches is not clear.

For those people who cannot or who refuse to take individual responsibility, public health practice may have to intervene and resort to a more paternalistic approach, for example, through policy and legislation to prevent the spread of an infectious disease, to protect population health or place an individual in practitioner care (even against their wishes) to ensure the well-being of themselves. Other examples are the enforcement of seat-belt legislation in motor vehicles and speed limits to protect drivers and pedestrians and legislation to restrict the sale of alcohol and tobacco to children (Baum, 2008).

Do health practitioners want to help to empower people or to simply change their behaviour?

Health practitioners have traditionally been involved with motivating people and trying to change their behaviour in an attempt to improve their health, regardless of their wishes. For example, the use of health communication approaches is based on educational and motivational strategies, as are social marketing and health literacy, to improve health. It can be argued that the purpose of most empowering approaches is also to change people's behaviour. The difference between an empowering approach and a motivational approach is in the methods used by the practitioner. If the method is directive, top-down and controlled by an outside agent, it is less likely to be empowering. If it facilitates a process of problem identification and action, based on the concerns of the community and using capacity-building strategies, it will have a much better chance of being empowering. Empowerment implies resistance and struggle to bring about a change in the political order and to challenge the very agencies that often fund and support health programmes. This can create an untrusting relationship between the funding agency and those engaging in empowerment approaches. The ethical issue here is should health practitioners purposefully avoid using paternalism and patronising approaches? If the choice of the community is not fully autonomous, or if it does not have the opportunity or ability to identify its own interests and concerns, then this enables top-down and paternalistic programmes to be used (Braunack-Mayer and Louise, 2008). Top-down programmes have been favoured by government programmes because they allow greater control by the practitioner and because they are easier to implement compared to empowerment approaches. In top-down programmes, it is the agency that selects the issues to be addressed, the implementation and evaluation, led by the practitioner. They patronise people who are managed and coerced into changing their unhealthy lifestyles into healthy behaviours. It is also a simplistic view of health and one that does not take into account that both individual and collective health is influenced by complex socio-political, cultural and economic factors.

A bottom-up approach

Bottom-up approaches are an alternative to the more predominant and coercive style of top-down programming. The approach leads to greater autonomous choice through the building of capacity, the exercise of control and the opportunity for healthier living (Braunack-Mayer and Louise, 2008). The way in which an issue is to be defined and addressed by a community, pressure group or other form of social collectivism is fundamental to its success. Adopting a 'bottom-up' approach helps the community identify its own problems, solutions and actions to address an issue. In a bottom-up approach, the significance of the role of the health practitioner is how they enable others to achieve this because at the heart of this approach is empowerment.

Government agencies in particular have to understand that engaging with communities is important because it provides the conditions for people to find a 'voice' when others cannot or will not act on their behalf. People that feel they have suffered an injustice or an inequality are much more likely to resort to activism against those in authority because they in turn create or contribute to the conditions that lead to their miserable circumstances. A major step is to identify and include the individuals, groups and communities who share an interest in the focus of the engagement. Participation is basic to community engagement because it allows people to become involved in activities which influence their lives and health. The engagement should aim to build community capacity to enable people to make decisions for themselves and to take appropriate actions. The identification of needs, solutions and actions can then be carried out by the community that in turn is much more likely to be committed because they have a sense of ownership in regard to the issues being addressed. Engaging with people is therefore crucial but it is not straightforward. For example, research in the UK has shown that of 80 per cent of people who claimed to want to get involved in public services when further questioned only 25 per cent were actually prepared to give up their time (Confederation of British Industry, 2006). Programmes will be more successful if they can maintain a high level of engagement, participation and motivation of people to address local concerns and is especially important when working with those low on the social gradient such as ethnic minorities, indigenous people and low socio-economic groups.

The criteria for the success of bottom-up approaches include: a small scale; a geographical locality, for example, the family; informal social groups and community-based organisations; implementation through NGOs rather than state bureaucracies; and the use of a flexible and participatory methodology. The potential advantages of bottom-up approaches are greater participation, community ownership and sustainability (Laverack, 2004) and people experiencing greater control over their lives. But to achieve these ends, the community must also be able to mobilise around particular issues that are relevant and important to their lives, issues which they have themselves identified. Communities innately take into account the broader underlying causes of powerlessness centred on local problems such as poor housing and unemployment (Kashefi and Mort, 2004).

While there are many methodologies for mapping individual and community problems for increased participation (Rifkin and Pridmore, 2001), the following is an innovative approach that has achieved some success.

Grounded citizens' juries

The **grounded citizens' jury** is an approach for local involvement in health decision making. Similar models to the grounded citizens' juries have been trialled in the USA and Germany (Stewart et al., 1995). What is different about this approach is that it can be used as a 'grounded' tool for activism in which local people are the agents in the development of policies directly affecting their lives. Grounded citizens' juries have been used as a grass-roots health needs assessment, for example, the concerns identified by people in South West Burnley, UK using this approach were as follows:

- low pay;
- poor housing and an increasing number of empty and derelict properties;
- increasing alcohol abuse by children;
- high crime levels, especially drug-related burglaries;
- poor access to health and social services;
- low literacy levels;
- teenage pregnancies;
- high volume of fast moving traffic and accidents;
- fear and mistrust of others in the community. (Kashefi and Mort, 2004)

The process begins when a steering committee selects 12–16 citizens to form the jury. These jury members are selected because they can offer an opinion on the health needs of their community and not because they represent a particular section or organisation. For example, jury members may be single mothers, the elderly, unemployed or people from an average family with children. The jury meets for a 4–5 day period with the purpose of reaching a 'verdict' on a particular long-standing problem regarding local circumstances and service provision related to the health needs of its citizens. The jury is asked a general question such as 'What would improve the health and well-being of residents in your community?' It undergoes a period of training in preparation for the meeting and is given time to ask questions about roles and responsibilities. It hears the testimonies from local health and welfare workers to increase its knowledge. Members are presented with the results of data collected about community opinions such as focus groups with school children and may meet with local community groups before further deliberation and the preparation of a report. The commissioning agency is committed to respond and take action on the recommendations made by the jury. The jury members are not practitioners or researchers and their deliberations can result in many recommendations that cover pertinent local concerns. Prioritisation is therefore an important step in focusing the jury onto a few key problems and the solutions that they are able to recommend such as improved service provision. The experience of being a juror can change the way in which people view themselves and their role in the community and can lead to individuals taking further action or in forming local action groups. However, a key point is the follow-up to the jury recommendations by the steering committee and the inclusion of jury members in this process of further development. Influencing policy at a local level involves a long-term community commitment and concerted and intelligent strategies for empowerment and health activism.

Lay epidemiology and health activism

Lay epidemiology is a term that has been widely used to describe the processes by which people in their everyday life understand and interpret risks (Allmark and Tod, 2006), including risks to their health and well-being. To reach conclusions about the risks, they access information from a variety of sources including the mass media, the internet, friends and family. Lay epidemiology can be an empowering experience for ordinary people and can help them to challenge the accepted 'wisdom' of health professionals:

1. People through reaching their conclusions do not necessarily accept health messages. People have recognised that some health messages are 'half truths' that can also change, for example, in regard to safe limits for alcohol consumption. Practitioners have chosen to use simple messaging that does not tell the whole truth by exaggerating the risks of a particular behaviour or the benefits of changing that behaviour. The prevention paradox is that targeting the behaviour of the majority who are at a low to medium risk has little effect at the individual level. For example, reducing dietary fat consumption for the whole population would reduce coronary heart disease but it is difficult to change the behaviour of those whose risk is only low to medium. However, an over reliance on health education approaches has led to mistrust by the public – people feel that risk does not apply to them, and they reject the advice (Hunt and Emslie, 2001).
2. People have cultural and personal values that undermine the meaning of health messages. For example, a person may choose not to give up smoking simply because it may be damaging to their health when they believe that the benefits of smoking, such as for pleasure or to reduce stress, outweigh the risk.
3. People can view any particular health behaviour in at least three ways: first, it is bad because it is poisonous; second, it is bad but desirable such as smoking; third, it is bad in some ways but good in others such as consuming alcohol. People's perception of risk therefore depends on their circumstances, culture and values and an 'all things considered' approach is taken. This is in contrast to traditional epidemiology which is purely empirical (Allmark and Tod, 2006).

Lay epidemiology is the basis for many empowerment approaches. Communities are influenced by the information that they receive, sometimes from many conflicting sources, and that they feel can place them at risk. For example, in the UK, public concerns were raised about the measles, mumps and rubella vaccine. The public health authorities saw this as an effective option with few side effects. However, following media reports of conflicting scientific evidence, the public became increasingly concerned that the vaccine could lead to bowel cancer and autism. These concerns were confounded by the past distrust between the authorities and the public over the handling of 'mad cow disease' and conflicting evidence on the benefits of screening, for example, for breast cancer using mammography (Smith, 2002).

Box 3.2   The Tuskegee study

The Tuskegee study was conducted by the US public health service between 1932 and 1972 and involved 500 black sharecroppers and men with untreated syphilis to document the course of the disease. The men were not told that they had syphilis, and did not receive any counselling or treatment for the disease even though penicillin had been an effective drug since 1943. The study was brought to a halt under pressure from concerned researchers, but after an expert panel meeting it was allowed to continue to allow autopsies to be carried out. Eventually, those concerned went to the press and a media scandal ensued which brought the study to an end. The legacy has been that black and ethnic-minority people have a mistrust of the medical profession which can act as a serious barrier to on-going clinical research projects (Cwikel, 2006).

In contrast to lay epidemiology, social epidemiology provides a measure of the well-being of populations, documenting and establishing trends based on its 'expert' and 'legitimate' power. Social epidemiology is the systematic study of health, well-being, social conditions or problems and diseases and their determinants, using epidemiology and social science methods to develop interventions, programmes and policies that can lead to a reduction in any adverse impact on populations (Cwikel, 2006). Social epidemiology emphasises that it is the study, by qualified researchers, of social problems in combination with epidemiology linked to the health status of populations. This sets standards of 'normality' that can be compared in relation to other population groups. In this way, health practice can build upon political concerns and create issues that they show can be overcome by using their 'expert' knowledge and power.

The Box 3.3 below provides an early example of the use of research to address an outbreak of cholera.

Box 3.3   John Snow and cholera mortality in London

John Snow (1813–1858) investigated data on cholera mortality in Soho, London using a new numeric method that revealed the rate was much higher in certain areas which drew their water from heavily polluted sections of the River Thames. His investigations in the Broad Street district were able to show that there was a marked difference in cholera rates when one company moved its water intake source to a less polluted section of the river whereas another

(Continued)

(Continued)

company did not. But when another epidemic occurred in 1854 his detailed house-to-house investigations provided conclusive evidence that the water supplied by one company to the Broad Street pump was the source of the cholera. The pump was sealed to stop it being used by residents and the epidemic slowed down. Legislation in 1857 later required all companies to filter their water supply and a greater appreciation developed that environmental factors could have an impact on the health of the public (Crosier, 2012).

The point of view from those in authority in the health sector has historically been that they hold the 'unquestioned truth'. But in an increasingly postmodern world there is no 'truth'. There are different opinions based on different views and theories, none of which holds an absolute truth. Lay epidemiology poses a challenge because it does not accept the professional 'wisdom', which then is no longer the dominant perspective. Of course, the means of governing people is dependent on 'expert' systems of knowledge, science and empirical truths. This is the means by which to regulate how practitioners are empowered to control health care, knowledge and a variety of social problems that do not necessarily fall within the bio-medical sphere. The authority structures in regard to health are part of the power-over that the state has on society (Brown and Zavestoski, 2004). But attempts to coerce or manipulate the public can place lay epidemiology as a means for their dissatisfaction to be validated and leads to collective empowerment. Health experts do use their power in a coercive and manipulative way to influence the way people think and act (Lupton, 1995). This is not always intentional on the part of the practitioner who faces the challenge of meeting goals based on empirical, bio-medical outcomes and which the public may not be ready or willing to engage with. The danger is that those in authority can present an illusion of greater individual and collective choice whilst acting to hide an agenda that intends to control others to do what we as practitioners want them to do, even against their will. However, the public is open to rational discussion and practitioners are right to engage with communities to offer advice that is based on sound scientific evidence. Health experts can therefore play an important mediating role between those in authority and those in civil society by helping to shape their daily conduct through rationality, research and self-regulation.

Health practitioners and the agencies that employ them play an integral part in the implementation of policy through programmes, projects and interventions aimed at improving health. Next in Chapter 4 I discuss strategies that activists can use to specifically influence policy and the role of practitioners to use their knowledge, resources and expertise to work with these groups to help them to gain more control over the policy process. I also provide a case study example of a community collective that was successful in their efforts to change national policy in New Zealand.

4

Strategies to influence healthy public policy

Many practitioners recognise the political nature of health agendas and the importance of helping others to engage in partisan politics to influence healthy public policy. But having a policy in place does not guarantee that health conditions will automatically improve. Alternatively, failing to have a policy in place that addresses health inequalities will guarantee little or no change. Central to influencing policy is the role of the practitioner to use their knowledge, resources and expertise to work with individuals, pressure groups and communities to help them to gain more control over the policy process. Enabling people to gain more control over their lives (and health) is the essence of empowerment. It is important for practitioners to think of a community not just as a place where people live, for example, a neighbourhood, because these are often a collection of non-connected people and competing group agendas. At a practice level, it is more useful to think of a community as a collection of individuals and groups who have identified and share the same, or similar, needs and concerns (Laverack, 2004). The concept of community is discussed in more detail in Chapter 8 and next I explain the role of community empowerment in influencing policy.

Community empowerment for social and political change

The continuum model of community empowerment (Figure 4.1) was first introduced to explain how unequal power relationships can be transformed to achieve more politicised forms of mobilisation. Each point on the continuum can be viewed as a progression towards the goals of social and political action. The groups and organisations that develop in the process have their own dynamics. They may flourish for a time then fade away for reasons as much to do with changes in the community as with a lack of broader political or financial support. What is important is that capacities are being built and learning from its own experiences, the community is much better able to deal with a range of issues influencing its members. However, the strength of the model is also its weakness: the continuum offers a simple, linear interpretation of what is actually a more

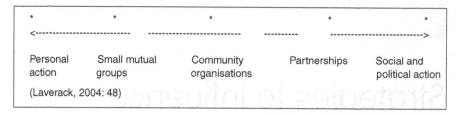

Figure 4.1 Community empowerment continuum

fluid and complex process. Nonetheless, the continuum provides a valuable tool to help others understand how they can become involved in empowerment approaches. The role of the practitioner is as a 'facilitator' to support and enable individuals, groups and communities to progress along the continuum. The desired outcomes are actions that bring about social and political change. Social change refers to societal norms, beliefs and behaviours that have an influence on the community. In turn, the political change refers to policy, legislation and governance that have a direct influence on the community. It is at the point of partnerships on the continuum when communities can have the greatest influence on policy through using their collective membership and resource base to take action (Labonté and Laverack, 2008). To achieve this change, health practitioners and communities must better understand the policy-making process and the opportunities that they have to work together to influence its development.

What is policy?

Policy is about taking decisions, setting goals and stating ways to address them through, for example, health projects, legislation, guidelines and codes of practice. Policy is usually made up of a combination of decisions, agendas and actions rather than just one simple decision and may extend over a long period of time. Policy can change over time and is influenced by many other factors, including other policy decisions and stakeholders at different levels involved in the policy formulating process. Health in all policies is an approach which emphasises that health and well-being are largely influenced by government sectors other than health and highlights the connections and interactions between policies from other sectors. By considering health impacts across all policies such as agriculture, education, the environment, housing and transport, health outcomes can be achieved. The health sector's role is therefore partly to support other sectors to achieve their goals in a way which also improves health and well-being. Healthy public policy covers a range of activities and decisions that cut across a number of different sectors, for example, housing, transport and employment, and that influence people's quality of life, well-being and health (Baum, 2008). It is different from health policy which is specifically concerned with the financing and operation of sickness care services (Brown, 1992). Healthy public policy involves a wide range of interest groups including consumers, government services, non-government organisations, pressure groups and the commercial sector. The competing interests involved in many healthy public policy decisions means that their implementation will often result in challenging the power of some groups who have a great deal of influence and wish to protect the interests of their shareholders, employees and members. And there are powerful interests at stake such as the pharmaceutical industry and the medical profession. Policy issues can be national, international and global and therefore can require inter-sectoral and inter-country cooperation. Because of the range of issues that healthy public policy addresses, for example, drinking alcohol, smoking and reducing poverty, its formulation and development is the target for many pressure groups, advocacy groups, social movements and activists, and is intrinsically a political activity (Draper, 1991).

The policy process

The healthy public policy process is complex because it is difficult to define the causal links between a policy intervention and an improvement in health. The causes of many health problems are due to the social, economic and political determinants of people's lives and there can be large differences between different groups, often within the same locality (Labonté and Laverack, 2008). Developing policy solutions therefore involves the use of a range of inter-sectoral strategies (Gauld, 2006), and sensitivity to its intrinsic political nature that should involve the communities they are designed to benefit (Yeatman, 1998). However, the people who control the political process (governments and governmental stakeholders at the national, municipal, regional and local levels) may or may not involve those who are influenced by the policy outcome. The policy process can be used to further exert control over people, resources and decision making, or to shape policies in the interests of elite groups to give them greater access to, and influence over, the political decision making process. In such an unsupportive political context, community consultation is not encouraged and empowerment approaches are resisted. Social justice and equity in society are undermined as is people's ability to participate in, take actions against or provoke activism against those in authority. Influencing policy can be a direct expression of collective empowerment, but more often, communities take conventional action such as voting, signing a petition or writing a letter to someone in the political system. However, marginalised groups in society often lack the resources or level of organisation necessary to have a stronger 'voice'. It is therefore necessary that some groups are assisted to become more active in influencing the policy process at its different stages of development. This is possible because, far from being predictable, the policy process can provide opportunities for the different stakeholders in civil society to negotiate a compromise (Labonté and Laverack, 2008).

People influenced by policy decisions may not necessarily agree with them and may want to change their formulation or stop their delivery. Communities can influence the policy process by persuading or forcing those who control its development to change its design or delivery. Public participation in policy change can take the form of 'direct democracy' such as a referendum that can be prospective and government initiated, or less commonly, reactive and citizen initiated. This is large-scale voting on specific questions often regarding constitutional issues about how people should live together and be governed such as compulsory military service

(Parkinson, 2006). Evidence suggests that people are reluctant to take direct forms of participation; for example, in New Zealand a study showed that of the 89 per cent of respondents to a petition only 19 per cent attended a demonstration, 17 per cent joined a boycott, 4 per cent joined in a strike and only 1 per cent were willing to occupy a building (Perry and Webster, 1999) to try and influence a policy issue. There is also a pattern of poor public participation that includes young people, members of ethnic and other minorities and those with the lowest level of education and income who are the least likely to be involved. However, some of these groups, such as young people, may be opting to use other forms of participation such as the internet (Hayward, 2006). Ironically, it is these groups who are most likely to be affected by policy decisions because they have less of an economic or social 'buffer' to protect them from changes in, for example, employment, housing or welfare policies. Influencing policy is an important form of participation that can be a direct expression of local empowerment, especially if people can be assisted to become more active at its different stages of its development.

Models of the policy process

Several useful frameworks have been developed to conceptualise how people can act to change the 'prevailing paradigm' of policy development. In particular, Lindquist (2001) offers an interesting view, provided in the Box below, of a framework to influence policy.

Box 4.1 A framework to influence policy

Types of policy influence:

1 Expanding policy capacities
   - improving the knowledge/data of certain actors;
   - supporting recipients to develop innovative ideas;
   - improving capabilities to communicate ideas;
   - developing new talent for research and analysis.

2 Broadening policy horizons
   - providing opportunities for networking/learning within the jurisdiction or with colleagues elsewhere;
   - introducing new concepts to frame debates, putting ideas on the agenda, or stimulating public debate;
   - educating researchers and others who take up new positions with broader understanding of issues;
   - stimulating quiet dialogue among decision-makers.

3 Affecting policy regimes
   - modification of existing programs or policies;
   - fundamental re-design of programs or policies. (Lindquist, 2001)

In addition to Lindquist's framework, a number of other models have been developed that, although primarily reflect processes in a democratic political system, provide in-depth conceptualisations about how this process works within two broad paradigms: rationalist and political (Neilson, 2001). The rationalist paradigm includes linear, incrementalist and interactive models as representations of the policy process. It originates from classical economic theory which presumes that actors have full information and are then able to establish priorities to achieve a desired and largely uncontested goal. It is driven by the production and consideration of different forms of evidence such as public health research, as well as the input from experts and academics as a valued part of the process. The political paradigm generates policy models adapted from political economy theory and derived from comparative politics and international relations. These theories stress the importance of agenda setting, policy networks, policy narratives and the policy transfer in shaping final decisions. Policy decisions, in turn, are made on the basis of bargaining and negotiation between the many different stakeholders who employ a range of approaches to have an influence on each stage of the policy process (discussed below). From the vantage of policy makers, the most effective approach to policy combines elements from both the rational and political paradigms. For example, the introduction of a policy to ban smoking in public places was initially based on strong epidemiological evidence regarding second-hand smoke. However, the best strategy to reduce death and illness from second-hand smoke would be a total ban on smoking including smoking in homes. Obviously, such a policy would be very difficult to police as well as creating opposition from civil libertarian groups. The policy decision was therefore a compromise based on the available evidence and the opposing interests of different stakeholders to reach an achievable goal rather than an optimal goal (Neilson, 2001).

A six-step strategy to influencing healthy public policy

At a practice level, the policy process can be defined as a framework that has six steps: 1. identify issues; 2. policy analysis; 3. undertake consultation; 4. move towards decisions; 5. implementation; and 6. evaluation (Edwards et al., 2001). These steps are subject to internal politics as well as to the politics of the state and the apparatus of administration and management that it employs. What follows is an explanation of how the policy development cycle can be influenced by individuals, communities, pressure groups and social movements, sometimes assisted by health practitioners.

1. Identify issues

Initially the health problem has to be defined and articulated before it can be properly considered and a decision made as to whether to include it on the policy agenda. Government policy agendas are often crowded and so issues that are to be selected are in competition with one another. It is useful if those people proposing the problem can demonstrate that it is an undesirable situation and one that is getting worse. In particular, they need to show that some public harm will result unless action is taken and that this harm is able to be expressed in terms of social and economic aggregates or health outcomes. For example, policy actions on obesity or smoking are more likely to be considered when the longer term social and economic effects, such as increased health expenditure and loss in practitioner productivity, can be shown. Similarly, the threat of litigation for economic costs, a strategy frequently used in the USA, has been effective to change the production, marketing and retail practices of food companies involved in the processed and fast food industry in regard to obesity-related damages (Labonté and Laverack, 2008). The responsibility to place a policy issue on the government agenda usually rests with the appropriate government minister. The minister has to ensure that there is a broad enough understanding and acceptance of the issue so that it has a good chance of moving forward in the policy cycle. This provides an opportunity to influence the policy cycle through indirect, conventional actions such as lobbying, for example, by sending a letter, email or text message, signing a petition or meeting with the minister. It is also an opportunity to influence the policy cycle through non-violent direct actions, for example, taking part in peaceful demonstrations. The media can also play a significant role and people can engage in a publicity campaign to try and influence the decisions made by the minister in selecting the policy agenda, for example, an issue that is obviously popular with the public may have a better chance of being selected. For example, Sweden passed a law against the trafficking of women intended for prostitution by making it legal to arrest the client and not the prostitute, an option widely popular with the public. This law came about through persistent media advocacy and the lobbying of organisations (Boethius, 2003).

But to what extent can public action have on defining the policy concerns of a government? Government action on policy can be seen as a democratic enterprise that, in theory, reflects the needs or wants of a significant proportion of the public. The public can express what they want through a range of actions, and can challenge the government arguments put forward for defining a particular policy 'problem'. The basis of these counter-arguments may be supported by research which in turn can be contested on the value basis of the problem definition. Inevitably, the success of one group's argument over another group's counter argument may be based more on access to the resources that enable them to put forward a more convincing campaign than the positioning of the issue in relation to the value of matters of public health, safety or individual rights. An important element of such a campaign is the media as it has the potential to widely influence public opinion. An advocacy truism is that having media coverage of an issue does not guarantee it will receive political attention; but a lack of media coverage will guarantee it gets no political attention. If governments are shown to be unresponsive to public demands for action, this can create the opportunity for others who do support the issue to step in and lobby to carry the issue forward.

2. Policy analysis

Policy analysis commonly involves at least three elements:

1. collecting the relevant data;
2. clarifying the objectives and resolving the key questions that have been raised; and
3. identifying the options and proposals that will form the basis of the policy reform.

An important factor is the level of investment made at this stage to ensure a thorough analysis of the issues and to provide sufficient clarity so that decisions can be quickly made to devise solutions to problems. But even when a policy solution exists, it may have to wait for a favourable political climate such as in the case of passive smoking. The scientific evidence against the causal link of passive smoking and ill health had existed for some time before it became a policy priority that was motivated from a position of moral and personal rights. This is when the 'window of opportunity' presented itself to act to introduce policy on passive smoking with the support of the public (Berridge, 1999).

Public health advocates, researchers (see Box 4.2) and academics can play an important role in helping to identify and provide the evidence necessary to resolve issues arising during the policy analysis.

Box 4.2   Research and policy

Alice Mary Stewart (1906–2002) was a UK physician specialising in social epidemiology and medicine and the effects of radiation on health. She was involved in a controversial and pioneering study of x-rays as a cause of childhood cancer, which she worked on from 1953 until 1956. But it was the investigation that came after her formal retirement, in which she and others examined the sickness records of employees in the Hanford plutonium production plant, Washington state, that led to further activism. Her study found a far higher incidence of radiation-induced ill health than was noted in official studies and that even very low doses of radiation cause substantial hazard. Her work on foetal damage caused by x-rays of pregnant women became accepted worldwide and influenced the change in policy in regard to the use of medical x-rays during pregnancy and in early childhood (Richmond, 2002).

One study (Haynes et al., 2011) found that public health researchers make a limited but important contribution to policy development. Some engage with policy directly through committees, advisory boards, advocacy coalitions, ministerial briefings, intervention design consultation, and research partnerships with government, as well as by championing research-informed policy in the media. Researchers try to facilitate the use of their work by providing scientifically rigorous papers. However, the academic language and lengthy journal publication timescales often missed the rapidly shifting policy development. Researchers also offered formal advice, making themselves available to policymakers for consultation and providing expedited reports and reviews, acting as research 'champions' and actively pursuing positive interpersonal relationships with policymakers. On the other hand, policymakers interpreted research-informed advice for inspiration and for pragmatic operational reasons, but they were savvy, somewhat cynical operators in a political arena who used researchers for their own means. This depended on the role and position of the researcher; the current stage of policy development in which they were engaged; the level of contention about the policy; and their assessment of the researchers' credibility. For example, high-profile researchers with a vision of their field and rhetorical skills were used to persuade ministers, stakeholders, and the public during policy agenda setting and formation. Researchers with a narrower expertise, such as specialists in clinical trials, were used to advise on intervention design and evaluation once overall policy directions had been agreed. More encouragingly, politicians and civil servants sought robust dialogue and creative thinking rather than policy compliant advice, and they valued expert opinion when research was insufficient for decision making. Policymakers supported researchers' views, in most cases, rather than simple researcher utilisation. However, in reality, policy analysis and development is mostly undertaken internally, and in confidence, and the level of invited public involvement and researcher consultation is limited (Haynes et al., 2011).

3. Undertake consultation

Consultation can be formal or informal and may occur at any stage of the policy process. Consultation is often facilitated by the issue of a discussion paper which outlines the policy intentions and allows feedback from individuals and pressure groups. People may be formally asked for a response to the discussion paper or it may be placed in the public arena to stimulate an open debate on the issues. The purpose is that the consultation stage will lead to a refinement of the policy and a wider public acceptance of its intentions.

It is at this stage that there is the greatest opportunity for 'legitimate' public engagement in the policy process. A number of indirect actions can be taken to influence the policy process such as attending a local meeting to discuss the draft policy paper, signing a petition for or against the policy paper or creating an advocacy group. A number of direct actions can also be taken to influence the policy process such as participating in public protests or by supporting a publicity campaign. The purpose of these actions is to ensure that the people involved in making the decisions are aware of public opinion for or against the policy, especially important when policy choices are strongly contested. Practitioners too are sometimes in a position of helping to draft policy and to convene consultations and can then be more critically reflective on when and with which groups are appropriate to include in the process. While the move to community participation by many governments is a potentially healthy step towards a more civil society, it is not always clear whose interests are being served most. Participation may have become a ritual, devoid of critical reflection on how it might be more or less empowering for the communities affected. In the end, bureaucrats become more empowered because they can say, 'I've consulted with the community, and therefore my conclusions have more politically correct weight.' If these conclusions truly do benefit community groups, this is not necessarily a bad outcome. But that may not always be the case and unless practitioners are clear on the reasons why they are engaging with communities on policy issues they risk draining their energies in discussions of no real importance.

4. Move towards decisions

Following analysis, debate and policy refinement the necessary decisions can begin to emerge. First, the decision will be made by the appropriate person and then the policy proposal will be put forward for approval by the government or the necessary body with authority. In spite of the earlier analysis and consultation, the final decision will have to consider issues of economy, efficiency and equity. A compromise may have to be reached, for example, one in which the policy is phased-in over a period of time to allow sufficient funds to be made available. Alternatively, the policy reforms may be introduced as a package alongside other measures, assistance and benefits. The purpose is to publicly introduce the policy reform with a minimum of opposition and criticism.

At this stage of the policy process, if people are opposed to the decisions, they can continue to use a range of direct and indirect actions: the threat of collectively withdrawing their votes for those making the decision, engaging in an aggressive publicity campaign or instigating legal action against those making the policy decision. The purpose of these actions is to try and force those making the decision to agree upon a compromise in favour of the opinions of those against it. For example, in Argentina, people affected by haemorrhagic fever successfully argued before the courts that the country's ratification of the International Covenant on Economic, Social and Cultural Rights and policy not to treat the disease therefore obligated it to finance the prevention of the disease (Labonté and Schrecker, 2007).

5. Implementation

Once the decisions have been made and approved the policy enters a period of implementation towards the desired outcomes. If the policy reform is clearly defined, has general support and is well resourced then the implementation should be successful. However, the implementation of a new policy invariably entails some modification to existing policies (Burris, 1997). Unless the implementation is delivered well and sensitively it can result in problems. Evidence from policy implementation has found a number of causes for a failure at the implementation stage including ambiguity in the policy itself, conflict with other policies, having low political priority or engendering conflict with significant stakeholders (Edwards et al., 2001). In particular, 'bad publicity' can have a detrimental effect on the implementation of the policy especially as decision makers often lose interest at this stage and insufficient resources are given to promote the reforms. On the other hand, the greatest likelihood of implementation success is when the policy is technically simple, necessitates only marginal changes in existing policy, is delivered by one agency, has clear objectives and a short duration (Walt, 1994).

Policies can actually be reformulated at the implementation stage and this provides the opportunity to interfere with and possibly stall the process of implementation by opposing stakeholders. The best chance of success they have is if the effect of 'bad publicity' can be harnessed against the policy reform. To do this, they may have to use technology to harness unconventional actions such as cyber-activism e-petitions; and virtual sit-ins or the refusal to pay taxes or to boycott the purchase a particular product.

6. Evaluation

The evaluation of the policy can lead to incremental revisions if reforms are not being met, or met efficiently. For example, if the purpose of the reform was to increase equity and participation in child support but this was shown not to have happened, the policy may be changed and re-implemented. The evaluation can be influenced by a broader political agenda which may also have changed since the original policy decision had been made. It may then be more difficult to justify a continuation of the policy if, for example, it now has a lower priority in the political agenda. Policy evaluation gives further hope to those who, if their actions and tactics to influence it have been unsuccessful, can use the revision process as a means to re-introduce changes to or to stop the reforms. Evaluation is an essential part of a cyclical process of design and implementation and allows information to be continually fed back to policymakers to adapt, change or even cancel policy.

The story of the New Zealand Prostitutes Collective

The NZPC is a non-government organisation comprising past and present sex workers advocating for the human rights, health and well-being of all prostitutes. The NZPC is committed to working for the empowerment of sex workers, so that they may have more control over all aspects of their work and lives. To achieve this, its aims consist of ensuring that all prostitutes are able to make informed choices to access services that will enhance their occupational safety and health and to work safely and in supportive environments. Other aims include liaison with government and non-government agencies and to provide adequate support to enable people under 18 years of age to leave sex work. The NZPC was legally constituted in 1989 when it registered as a charitable trust (NZPC, 2008). There now follows the story of how this small and relatively powerless group of prostitutes were able, largely through their own efforts, to influence policy in New Zealand and to bring about legislative reform in the regulation of the the sex industry. As prostitutes have gained more political and economic influence internationally, the term 'prostitution' has taken on a meaning of 'sex for sale by force', such as child sexual exploitation, whilst 'sex work' denotes a career choice (Ho, 2000; Lichtenstein, 1999; Rabinovitch and Strega, 2004). However, the terms prostitution (prostitutes) and sex work (sex workers) are often used synonymously.

It has never been illegal in New Zealand to offer money for sex or to pay for and purchase sex. Prior to the Prostitution Reform Act 2003, prostitution was considered to be a 'lewd act' but no penalty was attached to it. The sex industry was regulated by various laws including the Crimes Act 1961 that exerted control over brothel-keeping, living on the earnings from prostitution and procuring sexual intercourse; the Massage Parlours Act 1978 that attempted to control this branch of the sex industry (traditionally the largest); and the Summary Offences Act 1981 that governed soliciting (Prostitution Law Review Committee, 2008). However, although prostitution was not illegal, it was criminalised and prostitutes were effectively treated as criminals. The legislation on prostitution was approved by parliament, predominately a male institution, which mainly affected women, men and transgender people working as prostitutes rather than affecting the men who purchased sex. This made soliciting, brothel-keeping, living on the earnings and procuring sex, illegal offences subject to punitive action. The law had the effect of keeping prostitutes subjugated and subordinate by reinforcing a power imbalance between the largely male clients and female and transgender prostitutes. Male clients could legally buy sex and offer to pay for sex, yet for the female sex worker it was illegal to offer sex for money. What this meant was that if a male client initiated a transaction, he was supported by the law whilst the sex worker was forced into the position of submissively waiting for the client to clearly signal that he wanted to purchase sexual services (Public Health Association of New Zealand, 2001). In addition, the covert nature of massage parlours meant that prostitutes were vulnerable to exploitation, as unsatisfied parlour owners could threaten masseurs with exposure if they tried to negotiate better working conditions (Prostitution Law Review Committee, 2008).

It was the inequity in the law and the continual harassment from police raids on establishments such as massage parlours that 'triggered' individual prostitutes into coming together to question their rights as humans and as prostitutes (NZPC, 2008). In the early to late 1980s, the police could raid massage parlours as they deemed morally necessary. Because of the ambiguity of the law, the police could make up rules according to their own beliefs and then apply those rules haphazardly as they saw fit (Healy, 2006). Some police officers were more understanding of prostitution, whereas others were not and it was this hesitation in the law that disturbed prostitutes. An unjust environment of fear was created and what evolved was a situation that forced sex work underground. The owners of massage parlours were then able to exert much control over their employees, exploiting them by charging hefty bonds and supplying working conditions that were unclean and unsafe (Clarke and MacFarlane, 2005). Prostitutes in Wellington, the capital, who worked in the same massage parlour, met informally with the intention of discussing safer working conditions. The discussions first began in 1987 about forming a collective of people who worked in the sex industry with the aim of being able to gain employment rights for prostitutes and to avoid the development of an illegal sector within the industry (Healy, 2006).

The illegality of prostitutes was inevitable given the nature of the law regulating prostitution and would put individual prostitutes at an even greater risk of harm. Prostitutes are traditionally easy targets for discrimination which can result in marginalisation and stigmatisation (Rekart, 2005). Discrimination can lead to situations of abuse, coercion, exploitation, violence and low self-esteem, all of which can have a negative effect on the well-being of prostitutes (Cornish, 2006). Because of the laws that limited the freedom of prostitution and to combat the harassment and violence that a large proportion of prostitutes were experiencing in New Zealand, the NZPC was established with the formative ideal of empowerment: to enable them to take greater control of their lives.

This small group of prostitutes started to meet on a more regular basis in massage parlours, in the street, in pubs and at the beach. Their discussion moved to forming a union and to decriminalising prostitution as well as discussing safer working conditions. The shared interest created a connection that the prostitutes felt was unique and understood only by others in the same circumstances. What was important was that the meetings, although casual and without a sense of leadership, helped to alleviate feelings of isolation and fostered feelings of connectedness. By meeting and networking with other prostitutes in similar work situations, the group gained strength and a collective voice and was able to seek legitimacy through their contact with government officials, medical professionals, academics and political leaders. The group kept the focus inward engaging in peer interaction and outreach to other prostitutes using volunteer sex workers. This furthered their feelings of trust and helped to build their participant base as more prostitutes gained a shared identity and the confidence to challenge bad practice (Chetwynd, 1996).

The HIV/AIDS epidemic

A major factor leading to the official establishment of the NZPC was the threat of an HIV epidemic in New Zealand in the late 1980s. The government targeted three communities with which it wanted to form relationships to begin curbing the spread of HIV. These were gay men, injecting drug users and prostitutes. In 1988, the Ministry of Health (MoH) funded agencies such as sexual health providers and the Family Planning Association formed contracts with the NZPC to provide sexual and reproductive health services to prostitutes. This provided the impetus for the offer of government funds, infrastructure and services including small offices where prostitutes could access health care services, health and safety information and safer sex supplies. They also served as a place to network with others in the same industry and to communicate ideas about reform (Hann and Wren, 2000). There was a consensus among the members of the NZPC that people not engaged in sex work would not understand the industry and have difficulty relating to prostitutes (Healy and Reed, 1994). The members of the NZPC wanted to keep the organisation free from outsider involvement but they knew that to advance politically, the organisation needed to build partnerships and so they contracted a lawyer to help to establish a legitimate charitable trust.

A partnership with the Ministry of Health

Support for the NZPC grew and their collaboration with the MoH, along with the alliances they formed with other men's and women's civil society organisations, gave them legitimacy and a formal status. This led to formal requests for representatives from the sex work industry to be on various national committees such as the National Council on AIDS. The representation by the NZPC put them in a privileged position and one that allowed them to shift the policy agenda to also include the rights, occupational health and safety of prostitutes. At this time, no measures had been taken by the government to evaluate the current laws regulating prostitution. In 1991 the NZPC informed the Minister of Health that they could no longer continue their contracts unless a committee was formed to investigate repealing the laws against prostitution. The MoH conceded and an investigation into prostitution law reform began. The NZPC continued to raise the profile of the issues on prostitution decriminalisation by taking every advantage of media opportunities, developing posters with public health messages from the prostitutes' point of view, and by taking a calm, educated stance. Through their persistence and tenacity to adhere to an agenda of addressing social inequality, they formed partnerships with larger organisations that facilitated the achievement of their goals. But what gave the NZPC the most legitimacy and helped challenge the status quo on prostitution regulation was that it was in conflict with the New Zealand Strategy on HIV/AIDS (1990). This key strategy advocated the empowerment and enablement of marginalised groups. For the NZPC, empowerment was also a crucial concept that provided a rationale for their political activities (Lichtenstein, 1999) but with most sections of prostitution being illegal, prostitutes were being driven underground, a far cry from the empowering philosophies of the New Zealand strategy on HIV/AIDS.

Influencing policy

The NZPC actually made its first submission to parliament regarding the reform of prostitution laws in 1989, just two years after coming together as a group and around the same time they officially formed a charitable trust. At that time, the NZPC had close relations with leaders from other government identified 'at-risk' groups, the most influential being the New Zealand AIDS Foundation. In 1989 and 1990, the NZPC drafted submissions concerning the occupational regulations regarding the Massage Parlour Act 1978. This was perhaps premature because the NZPC did not yet have the support that they needed but it did help to raise the profile of the organisation. What followed were years of various submissions, changing governmental and other partnerships until the NZPC decided that a more 'political voice' was needed to champion the reform bill in parliament. Members of Parliament (MPs), allies of the NZPC, became involved and helped draft a revision of the prostitution decriminalisation bill in 1999. The bill then had its first reading in parliament in 2000. However, there was opposition. Some feminist groups and conservative religious organisations joined forces to draft submissions against the Prostitution Reform Bill in an attempt to gain support to defeat it. The feminist groups tended to argue that decriminalisation of prostitution would lead to more prostitutes, more brothels, more violence and more child abuse. The opposition by conservative religious organisations portrayed prostitutes as vectors of disease and depravity and tried to ensure that they remained marginalised from society. The opposition groups, whilst succeeding in slowing prostitution reform, ultimately failed at securing the required number of votes to stop the bill and never won over the public support they needed (Whipple, 2008).

In July 2003, after much debate, the Prostitution Reform Act was passed with the narrowest margin of one vote. The vote was a 'conscience vote' meaning that MPs voted according to their personal beliefs and values rather than following party policy. Sixty MPs voted for decriminalisation, 59 against and one abstained. It is believed that an impassioned speech by one MP, a former sex worker, and a Christian MP who openly swung her vote, persuaded other wavering MPs. With this narrow margin, history was made in New Zealand to decriminalise soliciting, brothel-keeping, procuring, and living on earnings from prostitution.

A study of the impact of the Prostitution Reform Act (Abel et al., 2007) several years later provided evidence of the achievement of both better equity and health for sex workers since decriminalisation, for example:

- 87 per cent of all survey participants have a regular doctor.
- Managed and private sex workers were less likely to report that they felt pressured to accept a client when they did not want to.
- Managed sex workers were more likely to report having refused to work with a client in the last 12 months and spoke of the support that they now had from management when it came to refusing to do certain clients.
- Few participants reported adverse incidents that had happened in the last 12 months to the police. Confidantes for bad experiences were most frequently co-workers, NZPC, a friend, or for managed workers, the manager or receptionist at their place of work.
- Most participants reported always using condoms for vaginal and anal sex.
- Clients frequently requested sex without a condom. Street-based workers were the most likely sector to report this and most survey participants reported telling clients that it was the law that they had to use condoms and over half reported refusing to do the job if the client persisted.

Since the Prostitution Reform Act, statistics for the number of prostitutes and brothels have also remained fairly static (Prostitution Law Review Committee, 2008) so refuting the accusations of those groups opposing the decriminalisation of prostitution in New Zealand. In fact, the evidence shows that the criminalisation of prostitutes directly contributes to violence, police harassment and an increase in HIV and other sexually transmitted infections (Rekart, 2005).

Those who formed the NZPC had problems and issues that were less rooted in their choice of work and their bodies than in the structured inequities of the law. The formation of the NZPC came about through the efforts of its members and the organisation remained peer driven even during the difficult stages of its development. Though it took 15 years to achieve a reform of the legislation, the New Zealand Prostitutes Collective was not only able to decriminalise prostitution but to form a framework that safeguarded the human rights, occupational health and safety of all prostitutes. Today, sex work in New Zealand constitutes behaviour between consenting adults and this makes efforts to enhance the health and safety of all prostitutes easier to achieve. Drawing prostitutes into the issue of HIV/AIDS and making them a part of the solution rather than ignoring or litigating against them saw prostitutes help curb the spread of HIV during the 1980s. Giving prostitutes the power to run their own organisation has resulted in improved partnerships and relationships with law enforcement, politicians, public health officials, and with society at large (Whipple, 2008).

Being able to identify 'champions' or partners, such as practitioners and politicians, who were willing to support their cause, based on a mutual respect and understanding, did help the NZPC. The choice of relationship that the NZPC formed with the Ministry of Health, a liberal and accessible political environment, and the timing of the profile of HIV/AIDS as a key population health concern were also critical factors. The rights of prostitutes are continuing to be strengthened through, for example, a further review of the legislation regulating prostitution in New Zealand. An individual's right to free choice, even if that choice is sex work, and the rights of prostitutes to have more control over their lives and how the sex industry is managed and regulated are important next steps in the future.

In this chapter I have discussed how activists can have an influence on public health policy. In Chapter 5 I take this discussion further to include the role that activism can increasingly play to address a broader agenda through the social determinants of health with case study examples in regard to unemployment, food justice and housing.

5

Activism and the social determinants of health

The social determinants of health

Health issues are often framed around the diseases that cause ill health and become further personalised by focusing on the 'struggle' against disease. In public health programmes, this is translated into interventions to motivate people to adopt healthy lifestyles and to change their 'unhealthy' behaviours. This in turn reinforces the importance of personal choice, personal responsibility and an emphasis on self-blame for one's powerless circumstances and poor state of health. The way in which society is structured, institutionalised and the inequities that this can create are not seen as a key part of the problem. Public health issues such as drug abuse, homelessness and social exclusion continue to be primarily viewed as problems of individual lifestyles. However, many health practitioners now recognise the importance of a determinant's approach in their work, one that moves beyond the individual lifestyle and behavioural model. The determinants of health gained prominence in the late 1980s are the range of personal, economic and environmental factors which 'determine' the health status of indivduals and populations. Addressing the determinants of health requires, in part, an approach that moves their work towards a model that posits health as being determined by how societies themselves are structured (Mouy and Barr, 2006). This has led to efforts to reconsider how practitioners can take greater account of the social determinants of health in their more routine work.

The health of the poor, the social gradient in health within countries, and the marked health inequities between countries are caused by the unequal distribution of power, income, goods, and services. The inequalities that this creates in everyday living include unequal access to health care and education, conditions of work and the limited opportunities of leading a healthy life. This unequal distribution is not a 'natural' phenomenon but is the result of a combination of poor social policies and programmes, unfair economic arrangements, and unjust governance. People who have, for example, high-risk lifestyles or who have poor living conditions are typically more influenced by economic and political policies, suffer greater health inequalities and consequently have more disease, premature death and less well-being (Wilkinson, 2003). Health status improves at each step up the income and social hierarchy. Higher income levels affect living conditions such as safe housing and the ability to buy sufficient good food. The social gradient in health means that health inequities affect everyone especially the poorest of the poor, around the world, who have the worst health. Within countries, the evidence shows that in general the lower an individual's socioeconomic position, the worse their health is and this is a global phenomenon, seen in low, middle and high income countries (World Health Organization, 2008). Prominent researchers such as Professor Sir Michael Marmot have claimed that social injustice and health inequalities are killing people on a grand scale because of the social gradient and the imbalances in the distribution of power, money and resources that it represents (Marmot et al., 2010).

There are four useful and empirically supported ways in which to model how social injustice and societal structures create health inequities:

- social stratification: where people are located in a social gradient (by economic, gender, racial status);
- differential exposure: to risks or hazards in the workplace, the community, the broader social and physical environments; the response to which is influenced by pre-existing conditions;
- differential vulnerability which increases the likelihood of morbidity or mortality when exposed to risks or hazards;
- differential consequences: both in terms of access to remedial health or other social services, length of time recovering from illness and the impact of illness on their position in the social gradient. (Diderichsen et al., 2001)

The degree of stratification and differential exposure, vulnerability and consequences are very much a function of economic and political policies chosen by different states. Amongst high-income states, those favouring a more 'liberal' (or neo-liberal) political economy (primarily the 'Anglo-American' nations of the UK, Ireland, USA, Canada, Australia and Aotearoa/New Zealand) have given lower priority to policies aimed at social spending than have social democratic states, for example, in the Nordic countries (Labonté and Laverack, 2008). Social injustice manifests across civil society and reflects unequal differences in the wealth and power of people. Those people who are already disenfranchised are further disadvantaged with respect to their health and freedom (Sen, 1999; World Health Organization, 2008). Any serious effort to reduce social injustice and health inequities must therefore involve changing the distribution of power within society, empowering individuals and groups to represent strongly and effectively their needs and interests and, in so doing, to challenge and change the unfair distribution of social resources. Empowerment is critical to gain the fairer distribution of essential material and social goods among population groups, through bottom-up approaches by those who are disadvantaged in society. However, the process of organising people to empower themselves to take action on health inequities cannot be separated from the responsibility of the state to guarantee a comprehensive set of rights and to ensure the fair distribution of resources among population groups (World Health Organization, 2008).

The 'social determinants of health' therefore encompass the economic and social conditions that influence the health of individuals, communities and populations. They are influences that may seem distant to an individual or community, but that nonetheless exert enormous influence over their everyday lives. The social determinants of health are the conditions in which people are born, grow, live, work and age, circumstances that are shaped by the distribution of money, power and resources and which are themselves influenced by policy choices (World Health Organization, 2008).

The Commission on Social Determinants of Health (CSDH) was established in 2005 to provide advice on how to reduce health inequalities and its final report contained three overarching recommendations (World Health Organization, 2008):

1. Tackle the inequitable distribution of power, money and resources

The key to addressing the determinants of and inequalities in health is through the redistribution of power and by transforming unequal power relationships which are indicative of our society and working practices. Inequity in the conditions of daily living is shaped by deeper social structures and processes. The inequity is produced by social norms, policies and practices that tolerate or actually promote unfair distribution of and access to power, wealth and other necessary social resources.

2. Measure and understand the problem and assess the impact of action

Action on the social determinants of health will be more effective if basic data systems, including vital registration and routine monitoring of health inequity and the social determinants of health, are put in place so that more effective policies, systems and programmes can be developed. While the central role of government and the public sector in taking action is necessary there is also a need for support and action in global institutions and agencies, governments, civil society, research and the private sector. The CSDH called for coherence between sectors in policy making and action to achieve improvements in health equity. Underpinning this is an empowered public sector, based on principles of justice, participation, and collaboration and actions including: policy coherence across government; strengthening action for equity and finance; and measurement, evaluation, and training.

3. Improve daily living conditions

Improving daily living conditions through the social determinants of health is an integral part of health programmes and an essential requirement for most people suffering poverty and powerlessness. The inequities in how society is organised mean that the freedom to enjoy good health is unequally distributed between and within societies. This inequity is seen in the conditions of early childhood and schooling, the nature of employment and working conditions, the physical form of the built environment and the quality of the natural environment in which people reside. Depending on the nature of these environments, different groups will have different experiences of material conditions, social support, and opportunity, which make them more or less likely to suffer poorer health.

Daily living conditions can be improved through actions to strengthen the social determinants of health, for example, where we live affects our health and lives. The daily conditions in which people live have a strong influence on health equity. Access to quality housing and clean water and sanitation are human rights. Broad policy interventions related to healthy urbanisation include stimulation of job creation, land tenure and land-use policy, transportation, sustainable urban development, social protection, settlement policies, slum upgrading and better security. Employment and working conditions have powerful effects on health equity. When these are good, they can provide financial security, social status, personal development, social relations and self-esteem, and protection from physical and psychosocial illness. The health of workers and their families will ultimately be improved by strengthening fair access to employment. A good diet and an adequate supply of food, for example, are basic but important to health and well-being. A poor diet can cause malnutrition and a variety of deficiencies that can contribute to, for example, cancer and diabetes and can also lead to obesity. Poor diet is often associated with people who are socially and economically disadvantaged (World Health Organization, 2008).

Activism and the social determinants of health

A focus on the social determinants of health provides activists with opportunities to address inequities in health and provides a guide to the specific areas where people's lives can be influenced by policies. The following is an account of three areas in which activism has been used to address inequities in daily living conditions: the insecurity caused by unemployment; the need for good nutrition and the need for better housing. I have chosen these examples because they represent issues that can directly affect people's daily lives, especially through policy implementation, but that can also be influenced through the direct actions of those people whose lives are influenced.

Employment and health

Job security increases health, whereas unemployment or the possibility of losing one's job causes more illness and premature death. Whilst having a job is generally healthier than not having one, stress in the workplace can also increase the risk of ill health. This is more pronounced when people have little opportunity to use their skills and have low decision making authority. People who are worried, anxious and unable to cope psychologically suffer from stress that over long periods of time can damage their health. For example, stress can cause high blood pressure, stroke, depression and may lead to premature death. It can result from many different circumstances in a person's life but the lower people are in the social gradient the more common these problems are (Wilkinson, 2003). One systematic review, for example, of employment and health outcomes found a relationship between temporary employment and increased psychological morbidity. Temporary employment was also associated with a higher risk of occupational injuries and lower sickness absence rates than permanent employment. The relationship between temporary employment and increased psychological morbidity may reflect the adverse effect of job insecurity on mental health. The higher risk of occupational injuries among temporary employees may be related to their greater inexperience and lack of induction and safety training at work. A lower sickness absence rate among temporary workers may be related to the insecure position they have in the labour market and sickness presenteeism, working while ill, due to a fear of job loss (Virtanen et al., 2005).

The eight-hour-day movement

The eight-hour-day movement was a focused mobilisation of the American labour markets in the nineteenth and early twentieth centuries to reduce the length of the working day to eight hours. The eight-hour day was a central tenet of all working-class organising and written into all working-class manifestos. Eight hours was more than simply an economic issue. It was a moral issue that embraced their beliefs about work, leisure, education, and health in the new industrial order. In 1864, the National Labour Union in the USA was established as a federation of skilled trades with the central goal of establishing a federal law mandating an eight-hour day for all workers. In 1867, Illinois was the first state to enact an eight-hour law, following two years of mobilisation by workers. American workers were divided in the 1870s and 1880s over the best strategies for achieving the eight-hour day. Some believed that electing labour-friendly politicians would ensure that their goals were enforced. Socialist and anarchist labour organisations advocated strikes to force employers to concede eight hours but saw shorter workdays as meaningless without an end to capitalism. Rank-and-file workers were more willing to use national strikes and boycotts against employers to obtain shorter hours. The national strike of 1 May 1886, succeeded in achieving eight hours for some, but was set back as a wave of anti-labour hysteria swept the country. By the 1890s, the American Federation of Labour adopted a new strategy of eight-hour strikes within single industries rather than nationwide. This strategy proved more successful and easier to coordinate. By 1910, employers realised that shorter working days meant more rested, productive workers. Public sentiment, too, was more favourable to an eight-hour day. Nevertheless, the eight-hour day was not universally realised in the USA until the Wage and Hour Law was passed in 1938 (Mirola, 2007b).

The collective actions of workers to gain more job security and better working conditions is also illustrated in the example of the *piqueteros* of Argentina in Box 5.1 below:

Box 5.1   Picketing for employment

Between 1996–2006, social action in Argentina was marked by numerous social responses to the socio-economic, political and cultural model that the administration of Carlos Menem had implemented in the country. Massive unemployment spawned a series of roadblocks that began in the interior of the country and spread to the capital, Buenos Aires. The roadblocks became known as *piquetes* (pickets) and those who participated were *piqueteros* (picketers). About 65 per cent of the *piqueteros* were women. The main purpose of these protests was to try and apply pressure on the government to obtain employment. As time went on, *piqueteros* began assembling in a more organised manner and forming unemployed worker movements. The picket movements shaped themselves into various organisations which developed into a complex network of groups with distinctive characteristics. Some joined political parties while others branched out from trade union organisations and organised themselves independently. The efforts of these organisations created additional pressure on the government to address the issue of unemployment and social welfare to the population (Di Marco et al., 2003).

Food justice movements

Food security is access by all people in a population at all times to a reliable supply of food from socially acceptable sources sufficient for an active and healthy life, in contrast to food insecurity when there is an involuntary shortage of food, often due to economic constraints, leading to physical symptoms such as hunger. Poverty is a major source of food insecurity. Efforts focusing on economic development as a means of ensuring food access, such as 'food banks', have been used to receive surplus food supplies and food donated through local and national food initiatives, to provide a wide network of food pantries and soup kitchens that distribute food directly to people in poverty. However, whilst addressing the short-term need of hunger, these interventions do not address the broader socio-political causes of food insecurity such as low-wage employment, mental illness, drug addiction, social stratification and declining government support for social programmes (Quandt, 2008).

Food justice movements have developed in a variety of forms to address food insecurity, quality and alternative forms of production or opposition to the use of, for example, genetically modified crops or additives in food. The collective approach to achieve food security proposes that enough food is produced globally to feed the entire world population at a level adequate to ensure that everyone can be free of hunger and fear of starvation. People should not live without enough food because of economic constraints or social inequalities. This approach is often referred to as 'food justice' and views food security as a basic human right and consequently has resulted in the development of a number of activist organisations that challenge the food industry and governments about the way food is produced, priced and distributed, globally. Policy coherence in addressing inequities in health is crucial. For example, trade policy that actively encourages the production, trade, and consumption of foods high in fats and sugars to the detriment of fruit and vegetable production is contradictory to health policy, which recommends relatively little consumption of high-fat, high-sugar foods and increased consumption of fruit and vegetables (World Health Organization, 2008). Food justice movements advocate for a fairer distribution of food, particularly grain crops, as a means of ending chronic hunger. The core of the Food Justice movement is the belief that what is lacking is not food, but the political will to distribute food fairly regardless of the recipient's ability to pay.

Like other cities around the world, New York faces problems of both high rates of obesity as well as hunger and food insecurity. In response, individuals and organisations have mobilised to advocate for healthier, more local, regional, and national food policies through collective action.

The New York City Food Movement

Current food activism in New York City is best regarded as an 'emerging' food movement with shared goals. The New York City Food Movement (NYCfm) includes parents who want healthier school food for their children; chefs trying to prepare healthier and more local foods; church goers for whom food charity and justice manifest their faith; immigrants trying to sustain familiar, sometimes healthier food practices; and food-store workers wanting to earn a living wage while making healthy and affordable food more available. Residents of the city's poor neighbourhoods also want better food choices in their communities and staff and volunteers at food pantries and soup kitchens want better food security. Health professionals are worried about diabetes and obesity and the growing burden of food-related chronic diseases. These disparate individuals and the organisations they influence constitute an amalgam of forces determined to change the city's food choices. They inhabit numerous social spaces, organisations and interest groups and exchange a variety of resources as well as varying levels of political and financial power (Freudenberg et al., 2011). Like any movement, members of the NYCfm have tensions in regard to their mission and agenda including:

- A focus on hunger in the city versus obesity.
- Community change versus policy change; the balance between alternative neighbourhood food distribution systems versus policy changes such as reducing federal subsidies for unhealthy foods.
- Supermarket subsidies. In 2009, New York City began offering incentives to supermarkets to locate in poor neighbourhoods via a programme called Food Retail Expansion to Support Health (FRESH). Some activists supported this effort, arguing it improves access to healthy food and helps prevent supermarkets leaving inner cities. Others claim that it fails to address supermarket promotion of unhealthy foods and lack of fresh foods, and that it risks gentrifying lower-income neighbourhoods.

- Cultural change versus political change. Some people join the food movement to change policies while others seek to build a community and the joy of growing and eating food with friends and family.
- Taking on the food industry. Food activists disagree about the priorities of increasing access to healthier food versus reducing the promotion and availability of unhealthy foods.
- Role of municipal government. Food justice advocates disagree about the role of the municipal government in the food movement. On the one hand, the mayor has played a leading role in initiating healthier food policy; without his leadership, the issue might not have been as high on the policy agenda nor attracted support from elected officials. On the other hand, with few exceptions, a top-down approach to policy has missed an opportunity to create grassroots constituencies for food change, making the changes needed to improve population health arguably more difficult.

Between 2006–2010 the NYCfm made progress in changing food policy, the creation of new programmes, engagement of new voices, and more favourable media coverage of food issues. Collectively, the NYCfm used a variety of indirect strategies including open network meetings, websites, advocacy and information sharing. The NYCfm played a key role in the legislative approvals of the 'green carts' (selling fruit and vegetables at reduced prices in low income neighbourhoods) programme which was opposed by local grocers, who feared loss of market share. The social movement was able to have more lobbying influence in the approval of policies because politicians were divided about appropriate actions. By calling attention to school food policies, regulation of food advertising to children, city food procurement and supermarket locations, advocacy actions were able to push for change based on public as well as individual and family opinions. The NYCfm moved food policy higher on the city's policy agenda and convinced some officials to make improved food policy a priority such as the zoning restrictions on fast food outlets, a sweetened beverage tax and purchasing locally-grown foods for schools (Freudenberg et al., 2011).

Food activists have also mobilised themselves to advocate for healthier, more just food policies to support food producers, as discussed in Box 5.2 below.

Box 5.2   Slow Food

Slow Food was founded in 1986 as a response to the opening of a McDonald's restaurant in Rome's famous Piazza di Spagna and growing public opinion against fast food outlets. Slow Food aims to support economic viability and supports artisan food producers and biodiversity through markets, consumer education, and political campaigning. As an international association promoting food and wine culture, Slow Food opposes the standardisation of taste and emphasises local or regional foods. It supports various local projects that aim

(Continued)

(Continued)

to safeguard traditional cultivation and processing techniques, for example, products that are threatened by industrial standardisation, hygiene laws and environmental damage such as yak's milk cheese from Tibet. Organisational units called the Presidia (defence battalions) are used to promote the products and guarantee their commercial future. The network of Slow Food members is organised into local groups called *condotte* in Italy, and *convivia* elsewhere in the world. Local *convivia* can be as small as a few people or as large as a hundred and also promote campaigns launched by the international association at a local level, for example, Slow Food USA set out to facilitate the exchange of machinery and equipment, seeds and labour to support small farmers who typically do not receive government assistance (Altiok, 2007; Petrini, 2003).

The housing movements

Urban planning that produces sprawling neighbourhoods with little affordable housing, few local amenities, and irregular unaffordable public transport does little to promote good health for all (National Heart Forum, 2007). Epidemiological studies have in fact shown an association between poor housing and health (Thomson et al., 2001) but the basic human need for proper housing and the relationship between poor living conditions and the determinants of health are obvious to many health practitioners. It is governments that create the policies that are largely responsible for the distribution of resources for housing. To influence broader government policy, it is necessary for residents, the homeless and activists to work with housing movements to gain greater access to resources and skills. Housing movements have varied greatly in their choice of tactics, effectiveness, and sustainability. Implicit in most housing movements is the logic that the private market is incapable of providing safe, decent, and affordable housing for the majority of those in need. However, whilst some housing movements are often reactive and exist for a temporary period, others have applied substantial thought and research into long-term visions of housing justice. Housing movements can be classified according to four main overlapping organising strategies: market intervention, construction of social housing, community control, and autonomous movements (Tracy, 2007).

Market intervention

Most housing movements involve some sort of demand for government intervention in the market place. This strategy pursues rent regulations as a method for stabilising housing prices and preserving working-class communities. Such intervention is favoured by many activists simply because it can potentially control housing prices in wide areas of existing housing stock at once through the legal system, instead of requiring additional construction of social housing.

Almost all local rent control ordinances operate by setting a price ceiling, or a formula, commonly attached to the rate of inflation, which determines the maximum amount of rent that can be charged for a given dwelling. In recent years, there has been some debate among activists as to the future of rent regulation as a strategy. Proponents uphold that it is a simple and effective way to prevent displacement. Critics have characterised it as a batch of basic consumer protections that will ultimately fail to protect tenants if the majority of housing remains in the speculative market.

The construction of social housing

Social housing is defined as housing that cannot be owned and operated for profit, sold for speculative gain and provides security of tenure for residents. Social housing can take a number of different forms including public housing, council housing and cooperative housing. The 'projects' as they became known in America were originally intended to provide government-owned, below-market housing for large sections of working-class people. In the late 1980s, the government of Great Britain started to wage war on its form of public housing, known as council housing. The developments were often demolished, reconstructed, and privatised, sold either to private corporations or cooperative residents' associations. The lack of on-going government support resulted in steeper housing costs and the exclusion of lower-income residents. This blueprint was exported to the USA where the Housing Opportunities for People Everywhere (HOPE) programme attempted to do the same. Throughout the 1990s, public housing was levelled and in most cases replaced with substantially fewer units. To preserve and improve public housing required determined local resistance aimed at city officials and bureaucrats. However, these campaigns often operated in isolation of each other and were therefore unable to promote a unified voice against the larger forces of displacement, privatisation and the destruction of the social safety net. The most common form of cooperative housing allows residents to own an interest in the building but their ability to sell at a speculative profit is curtailed and it is required that the occupied unit remain affordable to future residents. While many cooperatives are in fact unaffordable, many housing movements have used them to achieve their goals. Squatters have sought to legalise their situation through this model, and some anti-eviction organisers are attracted to the potential to take housing off the speculative market by using cooperatives. The cooperative approach complements organising campaigns where local control is as strong a demand as affordable housing.

Community control

Movements oriented toward community control analyse the housing crisis primarily in terms of decentralised, neighbourhood-based decision making in planning and zoning decisions. Housing movements often flourish when an immediate threat happens in the context of strong broad-based movements that forward racial and class demands. In Boston, USA many neighbourhoods in the city's South End were destroyed by developers and yet a movement by the

Emergency Tenants Council won the right to develop affordable housing. The development remains a working-class enclave in a neighbourhood that has become steadily more affluent and unaffordable. The fight-back against urban removal, and the demand for community control, led to the establishment of a large non-profit housing development sector. Activists sought ways to increase social assets and consolidate victories and many non-profit organisations have grown to administer federal and local housing subsidies. The 1990s saw an influx of young professional people into many rapidly growing areas in the USA and this contributed greatly to the escalation of evictions in working-class neighbourhoods. The most visible counterpoint to this was the Mission Anti-Displacement Coalition (MissionMission, 2012), which mobilised thousands of people against evictions and organised a neighbourhood-based city planning process. The coalition pulled together an unlikely mix of long-term, mostly Latino residents and newer, mostly white artists combining direct action with grassroots electoral work. In the USA, landlords recognised that thousands of units of decent homes would in fact break their monopoly on the housing market and were concerned that the increased supply would create a form of price control in the units that they owned. The most visible landlord-created anti-public housing organisation was the Coalition Against Socialist Housing (CASH). CASH and numerous other organisations successfully lobbied the federal government to largely restrict public housing access to the poorest workers. Through the clever use of local zoning laws, projects were usually located in ways that reinforced racial segregation. Throughout the following decades, public housing suffered continuous disinvestment, resulting in many of the developments falling into disrepair (Tracy, 2007).

Box 5.3 below provides a now classic case study of one group of residents that decided to take more control of their housing situation in San Francisco, USA.

Box 5.3   The Tenderloin Seniors Organising Project

The Tenderloin Seniors Organising Project (TSOP) was a 12-year initiative in the 1980s in San Francisco's Tenderloin district that used a community driven approach in a poor neighbourhood amongst low income elderly people. This group of almost homeless and destitute people living in single occupancy hotels had previously been labelled 'unorganisable' by the local authorities. The project's objectives were to build the competencies and leadership skills of the residents to reduce their feelings of social isolation and enhance social networks within the Tenderloin district. The project used three theoretical areas to guide its implementation; first, social networking (Chapter 9); second, Paulo Freire's (1973) principles of **critical consciousness** (Chapter 7); and third, an approach of community organisation in accordance with Saul Alinsky's theory that people come together around a shared interest to take action (Alinsky, 1971).

American social activist Saul Alinsky began to work to bring unity to the infamous 'Back of the Yards', a huge urban slum in the 1930s, a task made difficult because the area was inhabited by many nationalities. The intellectual idea behind Alinsky's work was to identify the indigenous leaders within the Back of the Yards and work with them to create a community-wide action group. Although this technique had worked in homogeneous areas in the past, it had never been tried before with widely disparate, ethnic and religious groups. The concept of community organising therefore came out of Alinsky's work and the key to grassroots organising was the churches, most of which were Catholic, and the creation of the Back of the Yards Neighborhood Council (BYNC). Alinsky worked to help empower the BYNC financially and politically. First, to be a 'citizen' meant that one had to participate in the community. It meant activism. It meant that people had to question decisions made elsewhere by authorities, and it meant being involved in larger events outside the community. It also involved learning the processes of functional democracy, such as engaging in debate, constructing bylaws and regulations, electing representatives, and working to focus their actions on important targets to change things. Alinsky wanted independence in the Back of the Yards but local politicians feared such independence and the bringing together of the disparate ethnic neighbourhoods over a common agenda. What ensued was a political battle for control fought out through media advocacy in the city's newspapers (English, 2007).

The Tenderloin Seniors Organising Project was initiated by a community development organiser and started in one hostel to organise a core group of elderly people who met regularly to discuss their problems of loneliness, crime and rent increases. Freire's techniques were used to ask questions and identify solutions and Alinsky's approach was used to promote social interaction opportunities to begin to address people's needs. Several other groups were established and over time, as trust and relationships developed, these groups recognised the value of linking with one another and to work on shared problems. The TSOP gained a number of 'tangible victories' such as organising a protest against rent increases, lobbying landlords for changes in eviction policy, improvements in the design of bathrooms to accommodate disabled people and establishing security of tenure. There were also improvements in health and well-being, including improved feelings of support, reported decreases in alcohol consumption and smoking, a higher consumption of fruit and vegetables and a decline in the crime rate (Minkler, 1997).

Autonomous movements

Autonomous movements avoid state intervention in favour of squatting and self-help approaches. European squatting was influenced by post-World War II over-supply of housing and enjoyed quasi-legal status until the 1990s with a crackdown on the practice that corresponded to the integration of the European Union. In England, Italy, Germany, and the Netherlands, squats have provided housing and organising spaces for anti-nuclear, and environmental social movements. The Lower East Side of New York City created a remarkable network of squats that included homeless, bohemian, and working-class people in need of housing. Perhaps some of the most spirited housing movements are now coming from developing countries. For example, post-apartheid South Africa has found itself in a crisis of evictions and unemployment due to the privatisation of many organisations. As a response, new social movements have emerged that use activism including militant style anti-eviction actions, rent strikes and eviction day invasions of courthouses to try and influence decision making (Tracy, 2007).

Communities and government agencies can work together to provide people with affordable housing and access to land for development and the Bangbua canal project in Thailand in Box 5.4 below is an innovative way in which this can happen.

Box 5.4   The Bangbua canal project, Thailand

Approximately 62 per cent of Thailand's slum population lives in Bangkok and 1.6 million (20 per cent) of Bangkok's population lives in slums. Nine communities along the Bangbua canal in North Bangkok initiated a slum upgrade project in the wake of a threatened eviction due to a proposed highway construction project. Through public hearings organised by the local authorities, it was decided that the people wanted to negotiate legal tenure and upgrade their communities. They worked with a governmental agency, the Community Organisation Development Institute (CODI), and an NGO, the Chumthonthai Foundation, both of which work within the national Baan Man Kong (secure tenure) housing project. This project required action on two levels. An operational level was primarily led by the community and a working group was established to coordinate the overall project. This working group conducted workshops and action planning with each community to develop the housing scheme and master plan. A network committee linked the nine communities and encouraged participation. Networks communicated with community members and gathered information for planning and implementation. A community savings group encouraged participation in a savings scheme that was transparent and included a community-auditing system. The CODI provided loans for urban poor housing and worked with other concerned institutions on land tenure, capacity building, housing design, and housing construction. The Treasury Department was the landlord and landowner and had provided 30-year leases to the participating communities. The Bangbua canal experience showed the importance of the need for community participation through networks that in turn allowed community members to engage in the housing development project, to build community capacity, and to assure other stakeholders of their commitment, which in turn provided the impetus in the process of securing land (KNUS, 2007).

Until recently, much of the literature on the social determinants of health has focused only on specific living and working conditions that create health inequities.

This has led to efforts to consider how health practitioners can take greater account of the SDH in their more routine programme work. But, unless health practitioners recognise the political context of the SDH it will be largely ineffectual in reducing health inequities. This requires, as is shown in the case studies in this chapter, engagement in partisan politics, empowerment strategies and health activism supported by strong civil society organisations with similar commitments. In Chapter 6 I discuss the role of the media in health activism and in particular I discuss the advances in information and communication technologies that have changed the way in which activists can operate today.

6

Activism and the media

The media refers collectively to technologies which are intended to reach a large audience via mass communication including printed materials, radio, television, the internet and mobile phones. The media offers an efficient and effective channel to reach both a large number of people or to target specific population groups. The media also offers low-cost options for communication as well as rapidly developing innovative methods with which to reach people at a local, national and international level. This chapter discusses the role of different media technologies in health activism.

Media advocacy

Media advocacy aims to influence the selection, framing and debate of specific topics by the mass media. In particular, media advocacy addresses the broader social and political agendas, rather than taking an individualistic point of view on health issues, and to influence policy that promotes health and well-being based on the principles of social justice (Wallack et al., 1993). The mass media continues to frame health issues within a bio-medical discourse, for example, access to treatment (waiting lists) or the need to change unhealthy behaviours. This is the perspective that gets the attention of policymakers. Media advocacy attempts to challenge this dominance by changing the frame. Social movements, for example, are constantly reframing the issues that convey their mission. To do this they must select the target group and set an appropriate agenda to communicate what is important. What is left in and what is left out is called 'framing' (Jernigan and Wright, 1996). Media advocacy addresses the determinants of health and the underlying causes of poverty and powerlessness, for example, unemployment and homelessness. It also addresses marketing, advertising and pricing in relation to products such as alcohol, tobacco and high fat/high salt food stuffs (Gasher et al., 2007). The goal of media advocacy is therefore to get the media's attention and to frame the problem and solution in an appropriate way so that policymakers, politicians and the public, understand the issue.

Media advocacy therefore targets policymakers and the ways in which issues come to be regarded as newsworthy to help set the discussion and to try to influence the boundaries within which the debate can take place. Hence, having an influence on what the media sets as its agenda can be potentially very powerful for advocacy groups. The internet serves as an ideal way for activist organisations to develop media advocacy relations. Understanding and providing what journalists want and need is as important as cultivating a personal relationship with reporters as it provides them with a portal for expert or alternative sources of information. However, one study covering 74 activist organisations (Reber and Kim, 2006) suggested that they were not using their websites to their fullest potential to foster media relations. Few websites included any sort of online press room or offered a site dedicated to journalists' needs. The study found that large national or international organisations are better at using their websites for press relations than small, grassroots organisations. Enhancing the ability of small activist organisations to provide better media information is an essential part of media advocacy. The study also suggests several practical guidelines related to activist online media relations:

1. Home pages of activist websites should include a link to a press room combining the information in one space and providing a link from the home page.
2. Websites should identify and provide contact information for experts in specific issue areas for easy access by journalists.
3. Websites should provide a mechanism through which journalists can contact the organisation with questions.
4. Regular email updates on issues of particular interest to the activist organisation and to the press provide a means of building an online relationship.
5. Websites should post news releases and updates with regularity and archive dated releases; and
6. Make position papers, backgrounders, and the organisation's publications available in the online press room. (Reber and Kim, 2006)

Media advocacy can increase a group's visibility and profile, and can magnify the importance of an issue. The extent and tone of the coverage has an impact on how the issue is then framed and perceived by policymakers. Media relations involve a regular stream of press releases when there is something important to communicate, such as the publication of a new report or a response to political events. Pressure groups will seek to have representation using the mass media including radio and television or alternatively, they may choose to hold a press conference at which journalists will have the opportunity to question the group (McGrath, 2007b). For example, pressure groups have successfully shifted tobacco control policy away from targeting smokers to targeting the tobacco and advertising industries. The tobacco industry had also used media advocacy to portray itself as a sound corporation providing employment to thousands of people and protecting the interests of their shareholders. The anti-smoking lobby on the other hand shifted to using media advocacy to erode the credibility of the tobacco industry and to portray it as self-serving, interested only in profit, irrespective of the damage that smoking can do to people's health (Wallack et al., 1993).

Box 6.1 below provides an example of how one organisation has been successful in applying media advocacy for action on smoking and health.

Box 6.1   Action on Smoking and Health

Action on Smoking and Health (ASH) is the name of a number of autonomous pressure groups throughout the world that has been successful in using media advocacy to achieve its goals to publicise and take action against the risks associated with tobacco smoking. ASH does not blame smokers or condemn smoking but instead uses an evidence based dual approach:

- information and networking: to develop opinion and awareness about the 'tobacco epidemic';
- advocacy and campaigning: for policy measures that will reduce the burden of addiction, disease and premature death attributable to tobacco.

ASH is a campaigning public health charity that works to eliminate the harm caused by tobacco, targeting groups and organisations using media advocacy. Its development has benefited activists from other sectors and using tactics that aim for political influence through the creation of alliances and coalitions. In the UK, for example, ASH is supported by the Department of Health, the British Heart Foundation and Cancer Research UK. ASH has purposefully established an international network and has moved into the arena of global policy frameworks. As a result, ASH has had some success, for example, in 2007 when it won its campaign for a total ban of smoking in enclosed public places in England including all pubs, bars and private members' clubs, as well as cafés, restaurants, and workplaces. A similar ban is also in force in Scotland, Northern Ireland and Wales and in a number of other European countries (ASH, 2012). The strategies that are used by ASH are purposefully indirect and conventional. Its status as a charity creates a dependence on funding sources including (directly or indirectly) from the government and this means that the organisation has to be cautious about attracting negative publicity through, for example, unconventional tactics such as media stunts.

Citizen journalism and the alternative press

The first so-called civic journalists acted as advocates on behalf of ordinary people and organised public meetings to put specific problems of local communities on the national agenda. As intellectuals and social movement activists entered the field of media advocacy the concept of 'citizen journalism' developed and people played a greater role in the process of collecting, reporting, analysing and disseminating information. The internet provided new channels of communication that helped to close the gap between the professionalised mass media and the public. Citizen journalism helps to challenge the dominance of the established media but it is unclear if this is because of the development of information and communication technology or as a response to public dissatisfaction with the system (Kern and Sang-hui, 2009). Bloggers regularly engage in citizen journalism and differentiate themselves from mainstream journalists by working through channels that allow them to send information directly to the public. However, some mainstream journalists also write their own blogs. A blog is a type of website or part of a website updated with new content on a regular basis by the user(s). Some blogs are interactive, allowing visitors to leave comments and messages and this interactivity distinguishes a blog from static websites. Blogs can function as a personal online diary and brand advertising for a company, commentary, or other material such as graphics or videos and links to other websites. Blogs are much harder to control than media broadcasts and as a result some political regimes seek to suppress them and to punish those who maintain them if they post 'offensive', 'anti-government', 'anti-royalist' or 'anti-religious' material (Blood, 2011).

The term 'alternative press' most often refers to non-commercial social and environmental justice print, internet-media, books, radio, video, film, and television. The term usually applies to sources of media that are critical, progressive, leftist, underground and dissident. The alternative press participates in indirect actions such as campaigns, conferences, or organisational websites where readers can engage in boycotts, buying fair trade products, e-newsletters, screening documentaries, writing letters to officials or editors and online protests. To understand why independent media sources are viewed as a powerful alternative, it is necessary to examine characteristics of the mainstream corporate-owned media. As media companies grew larger, they found it beneficial to interlock their boards of directors with other large manufacturing corporations, thus consolidating the interests of wealthy elites. Through purchases and mergers, the mass media became concentrated in the hands of fewer and fewer corporations, whose primary interest is maximising profits. This financial conflict of interest can create conditions for censorship, manipulation, propaganda, and disinformation (Andrzejewski, 2007). Corporate media and public relations firms have developed methods of creatively packaging selective information designed to gain public support for policies and practices beneficial to corporations and government collaborators. The alternative press offers another perspective, one that is oppositional and radical and serves the interests of competing pressure groups. Some characteristics most likely to be associated with the alternative press are: (1) committing to a mission that fosters peace, social justice, and/or ecological sustainability in some way; (2) giving voice to marginalised populations; (3) being a non-profit organisation; (4) critiquing and challenging misinformation and disinformation; (5) investigating, documenting, and gathering information from many sources; and (6) encouraging activism. The Alternative Press Index has been recognised as a leading guide to the alternative press in the USA and around the world. Alternative press organisations increasingly collaborate to support their collective goals and needs through groups like the Independent Press Association in the USA or the Independent News Collective in the UK (Alternative Press Center, 2012; Andrzejewski, 2007).

The mass media

The mass media is an attractive option to activists because it can be used to reach a large number of people quickly and cheaply. This broad-based approach can be used to influence public opinion, both positively and negatively, to lobby and to raise the awareness of people about a particular cause. However, the use of the mass media is not an indiscriminate way to cover a large, ill-defined audience as messaging can be used to target specific audiences in much the same way that it is used by commercial advertising to reach specific age cohorts, income and social groups. Individuals receive the information through a mass media channel but may also watch and listen with family and friends making it a social experience which can lead to discussion and action. Information received from the mass media can be quickly passed on through social networks, promoting debate and mass mobilisation. Some activist groups have used celebrities in the mass media to support their cause and to request for collective action or for fund raising events. For example, the USA basketball star, Magic Johnson, publicly announced that he was HIV positive through the mass media and later supported the cause to support young black people with the disease (Hubley and Copeman, 2008). Using the mass media can be more powerful if the issue can provide a human face and an authentic voice to the story. A quote from a prominent American producer emphasises the importance of this issue 'Acid rain isn't a story, it's a subject. Tell me a story about someone whose life was ruined by acid rain, or about a community trying to do something about acid rain, but don't tell me about acid rain' (Wallack et al., 1993).

Box 6.2 below provides the example of one activist who has been successful in using the mass media to address health and other issues.

Box 6.2   Activism and the mass media

Michael Moore (1954–) is a North American media activist who expresses his opinions through newspaper articles, documentaries, books, television shows and his own website. His documentary 'Sicko', for example, investigates the health care system in the USA, focusing on health insurance and the pharmaceutical industry. The documentary compares the for-profit, non-universal American system with the non-profit universal health care systems in Canada, the UK and France. The purpose of the documentary is to controversially raise issues about the weaknesses and inequities of the for-profit, non-universal system in the USA (Murguía, 2007b).

The decline in smoking in the UK has been attributed to the use of vigorous anti-smoking campaigns both by the government and by advocacy groups. However, smoking decline has differed between social classes and this may have been because the mass media campaigns were targeted at the higher, better educated and professional social classes. For the mass media to achieve real change, it must be followed up by face-to-face communication, with a discussion or debate about the key issues. The mass media approach must also be carried out over a prolonged period of time and may require a generous budget to cover sophisticated advertising campaigns. The use of the mass media works best for activist groups when their messaging is framed in a simple way, with a simple solution. The reinforcement of the mass media campaign from sympathetic journalistic coverage and professional support from, for example, the medical profession, will also help to increase the chances of success (Hubley and Copeman, 2008).

The following case study of the BUGA UP campaign targeted billboards to directly influence public opinion through simple 'anti-messaging' targeting mass media tobacco advertising in Australia.

Box 6.3   BUGA UP campaign

The Billboard Utilising Graffitists Against Unhealthy Promotions (BUGA UP) campaign was started as a response against tobacco advertising in Australia in the late 1970s to draw attention to the marketing of tobacco products by using humour and parody. The campaigners defaced thousands of tobacco advertising billboards by, for example, changing the slogan ('enjoy your freedom' to 'enjoy your cancer'), setting up parody organisations such as the 'advertising double standards council' and using a plane to sky-write 'cancer country' at a major sporting event. BUGA UP caught the public's attention and sparked several copy-cat campaigns by other activists but most significantly the efforts of the campaigners helped to change public opinion in the lead up to the national ban on cigarette advertising in 1994 (Chapman, 1996).

Community radio and television

Based on the concept that the airwaves belong to everyone, community radio and television provide a forum for people around the world to participate in social change. Community radio and television is a system that provides production equipment, training, and airtime on local channels so that the public can produce programming and broadcast to a wide audience. Community radio and television offers access to broadcasting platforms to encourage diversity, creativity, and participation in the media other than the ratings driven, market oriented, and privatised mass media. Community radio and television has been used by activists to focus on local as well as international issues using programme content that may be considered controversial. The development of community radio and television has been facilitated by technological change which has made media broadcasting and production easier, cheaper, and more accessible. Community television, for example in the United States, was assisted on a national level by federal regulations that were mandated as a result of the growth of the cable television industry in the early 1970s (Hackett, 2007). By 1972, the Federal Communications Commission authorised the creation of channels on new cable systems that would be available for state and local government, educational, and community public access purposes. Cable companies would be required to provide studio space and equipment that could be used by any member of the community to broadcast on these public access channels. Community radio and television provide a range of programming including talk shows, education and cultural shows and a variety of entertainment channels. However, they also offer the space for rebuttal and debate on issues of free speech, decency, and politics that may not be available in the mainstream mass media.

Community radio in Chile, for example, is considered to have contributed significantly to ending the Pinochet dictatorship in 1990 because radio stations that were operated by churches and political organisations provided information that would not have been allowed through official channels (Hackett, 2007).

Box 6.4   Guerrilla television

Guerrilla television began with the production of home-video cameras that allowed people with little technical experience to start producing video representations of events and ideas. It gave people the ability to decide how to portray everyday reality to provide an 'insider's point of view'. Guerrilla television asked society to question authority, not only the how and what of traditional newspapers, magazines, and broadcast television, but the why and who. In this way, guerrilla television can be seen as an artistic movement that asked people to look at the mass media critically in the same way they did other artistic mediums. Community radio, television and guerrilla television created a 'movement' that ran parallel with much of the counterculture of the 1970s and 1980s, of social mobilisation and activism (Stevenson, 2007).

Information and communication technology

Information and communication technology (ICT) is a general term for the integration of telecommunications, computers, software and audio-visuals that enables users to create, access, store, transmit, and manipulate information. The term ICT is also commonly used to refer to the merging of audio-visual and telephone networks with computer networks through a single cabling or link system. ICT allows individuals to engage with others on a broad range of social and political issues and also provides a safe space for activists' views to be expressed because they afford some anonymity. ICT allows health professionals to connect more readily with one another, for example, in Sri Lanka a series of progressive efforts since 2001 have used ICT to link health care providers with colleagues outside the country and to forge linkages among providers within the country (Edirippulige et al., 2009). Online users who engage through ICT can have important implications for democratic processes, for example, a gathering in which members watch a film helps foster a local community and provides an opportunity for 'virtual participation' (Rohlinger and Brown, 2009). The Queer Sisters, the oldest lesbian organisation in Hong Kong has used a virtual bulletin board to create principles, ideas, and feelings that challenged the status quo on homosexuality (Nip, 2004). The tactics available to activists via ICT allows the sharing of contact lists for quick and easy access, permit outside agencies to link activists across the globe and the creation of alternative news sources.

The creation and maintenance of a website can be an important tool for information sharing, organising and mobilisation to provide a profile and a 'face' for activist movements (Biddix and Han Woo, 2008). For example, Every Australian Counts is typical of organisations that are focused on a specific cause, sometimes for a short period of time, and use a website as a core part of their strategy with other electronic media to run their campaign.

Every Australian Counts

Every Australian Counts is a pressure group that has campaigned for a National Disability Insurance Scheme in Australia. The scheme will be a new support system for people with a disability, their families and carers to ensure they are better supported and to enable them to have greater choice and control. The campaign purposefully coincided with the Productivity Commission report to the Australian government on the findings of its inquiry into a long-term disability care and support scheme. The campaign is designed to lobby government and to advocate for change in the existing system and has a well-developed website that allows people to join online to contribute to the discussion and debate, provides access to campaign tools (stickers, posters etc.), materials, information sharing, supporter registration forms and links to Facebook and Twitter. The pressure group lobbies targeted politicians and other influential people and recruits 'champions' to support their cause such as media personalities (Every Australian Counts, 2012).

The use of ICT is rapidly changing the way in which people are able to mobilise themselves for mass advocacy, for example, through the rapid growth of social networks such as Twitter and Facebook and of the development of the Short Message Service.

The Short Message Service

The Short Message Service (SMS) allows the interchange of text messages between mobile telephones and is the most widely used data application internationally. It relies on Global System for Mobile Communications (GSM) access that is controlled by individual countries and whose approach has a direct impact on airtime costs, and in turn affects how many people have access to the system. The advantage to a government of a monopoly is control, not only business control, but also control over content. Information is automatically collected by the operators about the usage and location of every mobile handset. The capacity of the mobile telephone to organise people, record and publish images of, for example, protests, has already been established in the Middle East and in South East Asia (Banks et al., 2010). Mobile phones and text messaging, for example, played a crucial role in mobilising and organising people in the Orange Revolution in Ukraine. The Orange Revolution was a series of protests and political events that took place from late November 2004 to January 2005, in the immediate aftermath of the run-off vote of the 2004 Ukrainian presidential election. The election was claimed to be marred by corruption, voter intimidation and direct electoral fraud. Kiev, the Ukrainian capital, was the focal point of the civil resistance, with thousands of protesters demonstrating daily about the election result. Nationwide, the democratic revolution was highlighted by a series of acts of civil disobedience, sit-ins, and general strikes organised by the opposition movement. People took to the streets in angry protests and used texting to deliver regular updates on events. Supporters were able to simultaneously follow the events through social media including visual images on YouTube and photographs uploaded onto Facebook (Morozov, 2009).

Mobile telephones can also extend participation, monitoring and transparency, decentralise networks and provide opportunities for local innovation. The essential element is not high technology, but universality. Kubatana is a social and political action initiative in Zimbabwe that began on the internet, but to extend its reach it adapted 'FrontlineSMS' to send out regular news updates to people who had either no news source at all, or none that was trustworthy. It was soon discovered that the system was valued for its capacity to operate as a genuine information exchange, putting people from across the country in touch with one another (Banks et al., 2010). The development of internet applications into mobile phone systems has led to positive implications for e-health practice in many countries (Kirigia et al., 2005). In Uganda, for example, SMS has been used to improve community-based health care as is described in Box 6.5 below. While connectivity is still a problem, especially in some remote areas, it is improving steadily in most countries and people are able to communicate more effectively both with each other and with people who share their concerns outside their country.

Box 6.5   Mobile-health delivery in Uganda

In 2003, the Ministry of Health in Uganda set up a mobile-health network as a pilot project in two districts. The implementation was carried out by Ugandan workers from local and national health organisations and coordinated by a university-based research and development institution. The information content was developed through a participatory approach with the local health workers who were going to be the eventual users. This process involved the digitisation of the existing paper-based health-data forms, decision-support guidelines and educational materials. Technical support and training were provided continuously throughout the early phase of the implementation process. 200 mobile devices were distributed to 386 health workers and by 2006, 350 mobile devices were in use and a large proportion of these were used by community-based health workers (Iluyemi, 2009).

In a rapidly changing media environment, activist tactics have evolved to take advantage of the World Wide Web and the internet to communicate better, to organise, to mobilise, to lever and to raise resources for their respective causes.

Internet activism

Internet activism also known as cyberactivism and e-activism, is the use of electronic communication technologies such as email to raise awareness, to quickly mobilise people or to evoke a reaction to an event. The philosophy behind internet activism is that electronic actions can bring about social and political change through a combination of programming skills and critical thinking (Biddix and Han Woo, 2008). Internet activism, for example, uses e-petitions to send mass messaging to government, public and private organisations to urge for policy change and can reach a large number of people at minimal cost (Ayers and McCaughey, 2003). Change.org (Change, 2012) aims to promote social change specifically through the tactic of e-petitions. It is a web-based for-profit organisation that supports causes such as economic and criminal justice, human rights, education, the environment, health inequities, and sustainable food.

Internet activism can also be used in a more malicious and destructive way, called 'cyber-terrorism', a tactic that undermines the security of the internet as a free social and political platform (Samuel, 2004). Hacktivism is a more aggressive use of computer networks as a means of protest to promote political ends through the non-violent use of illegal or legally available digital tools. Hacktivists use a variety of methods to interfere with computers and computer networks such as website defacements by a significant alteration of content, information thefts, email bombing and the redirection of information. A virtual sit-in is an activist tactic that is conducted entirely online. Its name is drawn from the sit-ins of the civil rights movement whose purpose was non-violent civil disobedience. During a **virtual sit-in**, thousands of participants simultaneously try to access a particular target website, rendering the server slow or collapsing it completely. The goal of a virtual sit-in is to prevent others who want to visit the site from accessing it and is a popular tactic because the only action required from participants is to visit a website. The strategies behind virtual sit-ins have evolved from users crashing servers to using shareware Java-based tools, Perl-based tools, and scripts that can 'ping' servers so frequently that they are impossible to access. 'Anonymous' is generally accepted to be a term for members of certain internet subcultures, a way to refer to the actions of people in an environment where their actual identities are not known. Anonymous broadly represents the concept of any and all people as an unnamed collective using the internet or online actions in a coordinated manner, usually toward a loosely self-agreed goal. The Anonymous collective has become increasingly associated with collaborative, international activism employing tactics such as hacktivism, protests, petitions and lobbying. However, the actions credited to Anonymous are usually undertaken by unidentified individuals who apply the Anonymous label to their campaign or activist tactics. For example, a member of Anonymous hacked into the website of Britain's biggest abortion provider (the British Pregnancy Advisory Service) because he 'disagreed' with the decisions of two women he knew to terminate their pregnancies. He also stole database records containing the personal details of women which he later intended to publish. In addition, he defaced the website with the Anonymous logo and with an anti-abortion message. The identity of the hacker became known because of his involvement in a court case to prosecute him for his activist actions in the UK in 2012 (Leyden, 2012).

The World Wide Web

The World Wide Web is a system of interlinked hypertext documents, transmitted by web servers and web browsers, accessed via the internet. The internet is a global system of interconnected computer networks whereas the Web is essentially an application 'running' on the internet. Hyperlinks are connections to other related pages and to downloadable files, source documents, videos, images and other web resources. The World Wide Web was developed to be a pool of human knowledge, and human culture, which would allow collaborators to share their ideas and all aspects of common interests and needs (Brugger, 2010). The World Wide Web is also an important source of specific information, for example, a survey of over 500 users who went online for health care information found that 93 per cent were looking for a specific illness or condition and 65 per cent were looking for information about nutrition, exercise or weight control (Fox and Rainie, 2001). Another survey of 1,700 patients in the UK accessing a health information website showed a high patient demand for online health services such as booking GP appointments and ordering repeat medication. Almost half of the respondents (47 per cent) were aged over 55, indicating that demand for internet-based health services is not limited to younger patients, and over three-quarters of respondents (78 per cent) were female (Patient UK, 2012).

'Streaming media' is multi-media that is constantly received by and presented to a user while being delivered by a streaming provider. The name refers to the delivery method of the medium rather than to the medium itself. The distinction is usually applied to media that are distributed over telecommunications networks as most other delivery systems are either inherently streaming, such as radio and television or inherently non-streaming, such as books and compact discs. The advances in this technology have helped internet activism through live streaming, delivering live over the internet, involving a camera for the media, an encoder to digitise the content, a media publisher, and a content delivery network to distribute and deliver the content. A media stream can be streamed either live or on demand. Live streams are provided by a means called 'true streaming' that sends the information straight to the computer or device without saving the file to a hard disk (Lasar, 2007). An example of internet activism using streaming occurred in November 1999, when thousands of anti-globalisation activists converged upon Seattle, Washington, to protest against the meeting of the World Trade Organisation (WTO). A small group of activist technicians wanted to avoid mainstream media ignoring or misrepresenting the event and so they raised money and built their own open Independent Media Center, complete with computers, digital editing systems, internet connections and streaming audio/video. A worldwide network of internet activist sites, under the umbrella name of Indymedia (Independent Media Center, 2012) was created to provide an e-platform as coverage of the WTO protests, to spread information to a host of activist organisations and alternative journalists and stream their reports to audiences around the world (Lasar, 2007). At the same time the 'Electrohippies', an international collective, orchestrated their first virtual sit-in to coincide with the 1999 WTO and International Monetary Fund meeting in Seattle and amassed more than 500,000 people as an online presence (Weber, 2007).

Activists have turned to social media to organise people online and then for the activities to take place offline using networking sites such as Facebook and YouTube. For example, social media sites were used to help organise the Arab Spring in North Africa and the Orange Revolution in Ukraine. These social network sites have also been used to raise awareness about the purpose of protests and to gain public support for activist causes, at least until internet access was stopped by the government controllers. YouTube is a video-sharing website in which users can upload, view and share videos. Most of the content on YouTube has been uploaded by individual users although media corporations and other organisations offer some of their material via the site as part of the YouTube partnership. Unregistered users may watch videos, and registered users may upload an unlimited number of videos. Before the launch of YouTube in 2005, there were few easy methods available for ordinary computer users who wanted to post videos online. With its simple interface, YouTube has now made it possible for anyone with an internet connection to post a video that a worldwide audience could watch within a few minutes. Facebook is another social networking service and website launched in February 2004, operated and privately owned by Facebook Inc. Users must register before using the site, after which they may create a personal profile, add other users as friends, and exchange messages, including automatic notifications when they update their profile. Additionally, users may join common-interest user groups. Facebook has been ranked as the most used social networking service (Complete Computing, 2012) by worldwide monthly active users. It is available on many mobile devices and this allows users to continuously stay in touch with people wherever they are in the world so long as there is access to the internet. Facebook has been used by the news media to allow people to provide their views, live and online, in regard to a number of political issues and has been used to organise people in offline protests. Twitter is another online social networking service that enables its users to send and read text-based posts, known as 'tweets'. Users can tweet via the Twitter website to compatible external applications such as smartphones or by SMS.

In this chapter I have discussed how the rapidly changing technological media environment has allowed activism to evolve to take advantage of the availability of new developments such as SMS, Facebook and Twitter. This has enhanced their ability to communicate, to organise, to mobilise and to access limited resources. In Chapter 7 I discuss the role of the individual as an activist, the strategies that they have used and provide examples of how they have historically made a difference in public health.

7

The individual as activist

The role of the health activist

In 1847, the Prussian province of Silesia was ravaged by a typhoid epidemic. Because the crisis threatened the population of coal miners in the area, and thus the economy, the Prussian government hired a young pathologist, Rudolf Virchow, to investigate the problem. His employers imagined that Virchow would return with the recommendation then in vogue; a little more fresh air, a little more fresh drinking water. But Virchow had much more to say about the situation. He had spent three weeks in early 1848, not studying statistics or bureaucratic reports, but living with the miners and their families. One of the first points he made in his report was that typhoid was only one of several diseases afflicting the coal miners, prime amongst the others being dysentery, measles and tuberculosis. Virchow referred to these diseases as artificial to emphasise that, while they had their origin with a particular and naturally occurring bacterium, their epidemic rates in Silesia were determined by poor housing, working conditions, diet and lack of sanitation amongst the coal miners. For Virchow, the answer to the question as to how to prevent typhoid outbreaks in Silesia was quite simple. If you want to intercede you must start by inciting the population to a united effort. Education, freedom and welfare can never be fully attained from the outside but only from the people's realisation of their real needs.

To facilitate people realising their own needs, Virchow proposed a joint committee involving both lay people and professionals. This group would monitor the spread of typhoid and other diseases while organising agricultural food cooperatives to ensure the people had sufficient food to eat. Virchow's solutions to the typhoid epidemic over the longer term, based on his talks with the miners and their families, were even more radical, and included improved occupational health and safety, better wages, reduced working hours and strong local and regional self-government. Virchow argued for progressive tax reform, removing the burden from the working poor and placing it on 'the nouveau riche, who gained great wealth from the mines while regarding the Silesians themselves not as human beings but as machines' (Taylor and Rieger, 1985: 550). He also advocated democratic forms of industrial development, and even suggested hiring temporarily unemployed miners to build roadways making it easier to transport fresh produce during the winter.

These recommendations were not exactly what the Prussian government had expected. They had not hired Virchow to call into question the economics of the coal industry and industrial capitalism. His views did not fit within the mainstream thinking of ill health and he was promptly dismissed. Scarcely one week later, on his return to Berlin, Virchow joined with other street demonstrators erecting barricades and demonstrating passionately for political changes that they hoped would bring democracy, which Virchow believed was essential for health. He established a radical, yet prestigious, magazine titled *Medical Reform*, in which writers commented on the importance of full employment, adequate income, housing and nutrition in creating health. A decade later, still believing that political action was necessary for health, Virchow became a member of the Berlin Municipal Council and eventually of the Prussian Parliament itself. Throughout his 20 years as an elected official, Virchow campaigned tirelessly to get disease treated as a social as well as a medical issue. He planned and implemented a system of sewage disposal in Berlin and drafted legislation for proper food handling and inspection. He established better systems of building ventilation and heating and introduced the first health service and health education in the schools. Activists like Rudolf Virchow often move to positions within the state, taking their new ideas with them. Others already in the state incorporate these new knowledge challenges in various policies, declarations and state documents. Others may go into academia, influencing new generations of practitioners and creating new practice theories (Eyerman and Jamison, 1991). To Virchow, there was no distinction between being a health professional and a political activist. 'All disease has two causes', he once wrote, 'one pathological and the other political'. While he is largely remembered in medical schools for his enormous contributions to pathology, Virchow died believing that his most important work was the time he spent with the Silesian miners, understanding how social conditions can either create health, or produce illness (Taylor and Rieger, 1985).

Virchow's story tells us that, whether infectious or chronic, diseases are physiological events that arise within, and derive their meaning or significance from, particular social and political contexts. Virchow's story also foreshadows the important role played by educated, empowered and organised groups of citizens in creating healthy social change. Infectious diseases declined dramatically in industrialised countries at the end of the last century, a transition in large part resulting from social and political changes such as improved sanitation, improved working and living conditions, improved nutrition and family planning. These changes did not come easily. Employers often opposed sanitary reforms and quarantine on imported goods because they reduced profits. Working-class organisation for improved wages and better working conditions was often brutally repressed by elite groups whose interests were challenged. Gains of the nineteenth century arose from the entwined activist efforts of organised workers groups, women's groups, enlightened health professionals, activists and political reformers.

Rudolf Virchow is one of many enlightened health professionals who have played an important role in bridging the gap between the state and civil society and who have demonstrated that the 'professional should always be political'. The professional must recognise the political nature of health agendas otherwise they will be largely ineffectual in reducing health inequities. This requires professionals, and the people that they work with, to engage in partisan politics to influence policy and practice. This does not entirely guarantee that health conditions will improve but failing to have a policy in place that addresses health inequities will guarantee little or no change. Other activist-professionals who have used their position to work to address health inequities include:

Rose Kushner (1929–1990) was a 45-year-old American journalist when in 1974 she was diagnosed with breast cancer. The standard procedure at that time in the USA was to perform a tumour biopsy and radical mastectomy in a single surgical operation in which muscle tissue and lymph nodes were removed along with the breast. Rose Kushner objected to this very invasive procedure but could not find a doctor who would perform a diagnostic biopsy and allow her to decide what action to take next. Finally she found a doctor in New York who was willing to do a modified radical mastectomy. She was deeply affected by her experiences with breast cancer and embarked on learning more about treatment options and provided advice for patients, including criticism of radical mastectomies and the practice of performing a biopsy and a mastectomy as a one-step surgical procedure. Her rhetoric was strongly feminist and emphasised the right of women to make decisions about their own bodies thus openly criticising the medical profession (Lerner, 2001). Kushner established the Breast Cancer Advisory Center responding to calls and letters from thousands of women wanting information about breast cancer and its treatment. The centre's establishment was motivated in part by Kushner's desire to promote patient self-help and mutual support, thus displacing the medical profession and the American Cancer Society from their roles as information 'gatekeepers' (Kasper and Ferguson, 2001). Kushner was a relentless activist, lobbying, representing women on advisory boards and technical panels and attending numerous meetings of medical professionals, interrupting presentations, questioning conclusions, and speaking against the practice of one-step breast cancer surgery. In 1979 the National Institutes of Health (of which Kushner was a lay member) concluded that radical mastectomy should no longer be the standard treatment for suspected cases of breast cancer but recommended total simple mastectomy as the primary surgical treatment (Lerner, 2001).

Margaret Sanger (1879–1966) was a key advocate for birth control at a time when it was illegal for any woman, even those who were married, to use these methods. Sanger argued that women would not be fully able to participate in life outside the home until they could control when and if they became pregnant. She was born in New York to a Catholic mother who had 18 pregnancies, 11 of which resulted in live births. Sanger herself had three children, all of them dying in their childhoods. In 1916, Sanger opened a family planning and birth control clinic in Brooklyn, the first of its kind in the USA, violating laws concerning the dissemination of information for the purposes of birth control. The clinic was raided by the police and Sanger was arrested and imprisoned where she continued to give lectures to the inmates on hygiene and reproduction. Sanger founded the American Birth Control League in 1921 and in 1923 established the first legal birth control clinic in the USA. It was not until 1960 when the birth control pill became available to the general public and, in 1966, birth control was actually legalised for married couples in the United States (Randall, 2007).

Richard Cloward (1926–2001) and Frances Fox Piven (1932–), two influential American social reformers, showed that only half of eligible poor women actually received welfare benefits, and argued that the welfare system was able to function only because it actively excluded so many. They proposed to enrol all those who were eligible, thereby bankrupting local relief agencies and forcing the federal government to establish a national relief programme. Their thinking subsequently informed much of the welfare rights movement's activities and helped expand the food stamp programme, forced tens of millions of dollars in relief money to be put into the hands of poor women and to bring poor black women into politics as agents of change. Cloward and Piven also argued that welfare programmes were not benevolent efforts to aid poor people but are rather created or expanded only in times of crisis in order to placate the poor. When that disruption subsides, relief programmes are then cut back in order to force recipients into the low-wage labour market allowing government regulation of both civil disorder and low-wage employment. In 1983, they founded Human SERVE (Human Services Employees Registration and Voter Education), whose research and activism ultimately led to the 1993 National Voter Registration Act. The law requires public agencies, including departments for motor vehicles and welfare offices, to offer easy access to voter registration forms (Pimpare, 2007).

Harvey Milk (1930–78) is described as one of the most influential gay rights activists of the twentieth century. Milk started the Castro Valley Association, an organisation that helped the gay community become politically organised and gain allies within labour unions and local political leaders. After running for a seat on the San Francisco Board four times, he won the election in 1977, becoming the first openly gay person to hold office in the USA. But this victory would not last and Milk was murdered after he had served only 11 months on the board. Milk's legacy continued and 100,000 people marched on the first anniversary of his death to the nation's capital in support of gay rights (Shilts, 1982).

In this book I discuss the courageous and innovative work of many other activists who have historically played an important role in addressing health inequities. What individuals such as Rudolf Virchow and Rose Kushner have in common is an ability to facilitate the empowerment of others. Individuals do operate on their own, largely or entirely independent of groups, producing campaign materials and holding single-person vigils about causes that few others are willing to champion. However, people are most successful when they engage collectively, rather than acting as an individual, to change the structural and systemic causes of inequity through social and political action. Individuals achieve these goals through their involvement in social groups, communities, partnerships and networks, by mobilising resources, improving their personal competencies and by using a range of (conventional and unconventional) tactics. By operating collectively, activists can also gain several advantages. They can undertake larger tasks, such as organising a national campaign, can benefit from sharing roles and responsibilities and can also give a feeling of solidarity and provide mutual support to one another.

Individual activist leaders have the passion and courage to provide direction on issues that may not be considered mainstream, and may even be considered subversive. Virchow, for example, was not thanked for his activist views on the underlying causes of the deaths of Silesian miners. Virchow himself was further dismayed by how the poverty of the Silesian miners induced a sort of apathy or resignation in them and recognised that 'Inciting the people to a united effort' is not easy work. The resignation to one's fate and an inability to take action has been called the 'apathy of the poor'. It is a phenomenon (Lerner, 1986) that occurs with persons living in risk conditions. They begin to accept aspects of their world that are self-destructive to their own health and well-being, thinking that these are unalterable features of what they take to be 'reality'. Part of this internalising process is isolation, removing oneself from active group participation because of low self-esteem and high self-blame. Poorer people internalise self-blame for their poverty. Their self-esteem plummets and they isolate themselves from others (Berkman, 1986). Activist leaders are able to work with these people to build their confidence, competence and ability, to enable them to gain more control over their lives.

Strategies for individual activists

Oppressed peoples often produce their own leaders and organisers. These people often have a motivational and power-transforming presence that inspires and mobilises others in the cause. But there is also an important 'outside' role that individuals can play in this process, for example, Sir Edwin Chadwick (1800–90) was an English social reformer, noted for his work on the Poor Laws and the improvement of sanitary conditions and public health. In 1832 Chadwick was employed to inquire into the operation of and reform of the poor. In 1834 individual parishes were grouped into Poor Law Unions each with a union workhouse, although Chadwick fought for a more centralised system of administration controlled from a central board. While still officially working with the Poor Law, Chadwick also took up the question of poor sanitation. He was a commissioner of the Metropolitan Commission of Sewers in London from 1848 to 1849 and a commissioner of the General Board of Health from its establishment in 1848 to its abolition in 1854. In January 1884, he was appointed as the first president of the Association of Public Sanitary Inspectors (Chartered Institute of Environmental Health, 2012).

Enlightened health professionals and activists can provide a link between less powerful groups and more powerful public institutions, political and economic leaders and organisations. Individuals are most effective when they understand their own power base including the specific knowledge, financial resources and skills that they possess. They can also use specific strategies that enable others to gain more control over their lives (and health), in particular, critical consciousness; advocacy and leadership qualities for activism.

Critical consciousness

Communities cannot intentionally empower themselves without having an understanding of the underlying causes of their powerlessness. This is the process of critical consciousness and may occur from within the community, 'organically', or as an intervention driven by an outside agent. Critical consciousness is also described as '... the ability to reflect on the assumptions underlying our and others' ideas and actions and to contemplate alternative ways of living' (Goodman et al., 1998, p.272). This process of discussion, reflection and action has also been termed 'critical awareness', 'critical reflection', 'critical thinking' and 'dialectical thinking'. It is a process of emancipation through learning or education such as 'empowerment education', developed by the educationalist Paulo Freire (1973) whose original ideas came from literacy programmes in the 1950s for slum dwellers and peasants in Brazil. To Freire, the central premise was that education is not neutral but is influenced by the context of one's life. The purpose of education is liberation and emancipation. People become the subjects of their own learning involving critical reflection and analysis of personal circumstances (Wallerstein and Bernstein, 1988). To achieve this, Freire proposed a group dialogue approach to share ideas and experiences and to promote critical thinking by posing problems to allow people to uncover the root causes of their disempowerment. Once critically aware, people can plan more effective actions to change the circumstances of their disempowerment, a defining prerequisite in the process of empowerment. He showed that working to raise the critical consciousness of people with poor basic literacy skills can lead to outcomes that are closely aligned with empowerment (Nutbeam, 2000). This enables people to understand better the underlying social and political causes of their poor health and powerlessness and in turn can lead to people taking action to address these circumstances, including through activism. This is an on-going interaction of action/reflection/action that can lead to collective social and political activity (Freire, 1973). The approach does involve a considerable commitment to be able to gradually understand the causes of their powerlessness and to develop realistic actions to begin to resolve the structural conditions that created them in the first place.

Photovoice

An example of how being critically conscious can influence health outcomes is provided through the use of **Photovoice** by Caroline Wang and her colleagues (Wang et al., 1998). Photovoice, is a process that uses the work of Paulo Freire to enable people to identify, represent, and enhance their community through a specific photographic technique. It entrusts cameras to the hands of people to enable them to act as recorders, and potential catalysts for social action and change, in their own communities. It uses the immediacy of the visual image and accompanying stories to furnish evidence and to promote an effective, participatory means of sharing expertise to create healthful public policy. Photovoice can be used to reach, inform, and organise community members, enabling them to prioritise their concerns and discuss problems and solutions. Photovoice goes beyond the conventional role of community assessment by inviting people to promote their own and their community's well-being. It is a method that enables people to define for themselves and others, including policymakers, what is worth remembering and what needs to be changed (Photovoice, 2008).

Photovoice has two main goals:

- to enable people to record and reflect their community's strengths and concerns;
- to promote critical dialogue and knowledge about personal and community issues through group discussions of photographs.

People using Photovoice engage in a three-stage process that provides the foundation for analysing the pictures they have taken:

Stage 1, selecting: choosing those photographs that most accurately reflect the community's concerns and assets. So that people can lead the discussion, it is they who choose the photographs. They select photographs they consider most significant, or simply like best, from each roll of film they have taken.

Stage 2, contextualising or story telling: the participatory approach also generates the second stage, contextualising or storytelling. This occurs in the process of group discussion, voicing our individual and collective experience. Photographs alone, considered outside the context of their own voices and stories, would not add to the essence of Photovoice. People, therefore, have to describe the meaning of their images in group discussions and it is this that provides meaning, understanding and context.

Stage 3, codifying: the participatory approach gives multiple meanings to singular images and thus frames the third stage, codifying. In this stage, participants may identify three types of dimensions that arise from the dialogue process: issues, themes or theories. The individual or group may codify issues when the concerns targeted for action are pragmatic, immediate, and tangible. This is the most direct application of the analysis. The individual or group may also codify themes and patterns, or develop theories that are grounded in a more systematic analysis of the images.

Box 7.1 provides a case study of how Photovoice can be used to promote community action.

Box 7.1 Photovoice and resident action

St Jamestown is an established immigrant-receiving area of great ethno-racial diversity in Toronto. It is the most densely populated area in Canada with 64,636 people living in 18-year-old high-rise rental apartment buildings. Residents represent a broad range of ethnic backgrounds, including Tamil, Chinese, Filipino, Somali, Kenyan, Arab, Tibetan, Bangladeshi, Nepali, Pakistani and West Indian. The Photovoice approach was used to help newcomer communities influence public policy, secure improved local services, and enhance existing community strengths that promote health and well-being. Images of community issues were taken by people living in the area and then an account or photo-story was created to explain what was important in the picture. Using as many of the participants' own words as possible, short captions from the photo-stories were created. The resident action group displayed the images at a Community Forum and Exposition, attended by over 300 people. It was decided by the action group to next take these issues to the city councillor's office. The recommendations made to the city authorities were modest and related to day-to-day living issues affecting all age groups in the neighbourhood. Bicycle theft due to improperly maintained bicycle racks was identified as a common problem. Since cycling is the main mode of transport for many residents in this neighbourhood, safe bicycle storage is a daily concern for many residents. The action group worked with the city authorities to take an inventory of all bicycle racks, arrange the removal of broken bicycles from existing racks and install new racks in the neighbourhood. The decision of city authorities to remove broken and abandoned bicycles from the neighbourhood was as a direct result of the Photovoice approach. The group was successful in advocating for changes which required intervention at the city level but the broader issues such as employment opportunities, recognition of foreign qualifications, housing repairs and health care accessibility remained unaddressed (Haque and Eng, 2011).

Similar experiences of addressing local issues in regard to maternal and child health (Wang and Pies, 2004) and the concerns of adolescents (Wilson et al., 2007) have been achieved using the Photovoice approach. Having an influence on the broader causes of poverty and powerlessness, for example, unemployment and social exclusion have not been achieved using Photovoice because these require further political commitment. Photovoice is a 'tool' that can only help to engage community members in needs assessment, asset mapping, and programme planning and assist people to advocate for change.

Advocacy

Advocacy involves people acting on behalf of themselves or on behalf of others to argue a position and to influence the outcome of decisions. The main aim of advocacy is to help others to speak and act on their own behalf. Anyone can use advocacy but in practice initiatives are usually started to support particular causes, groups and ideologies (Smithies and Webster, 1998). Advocacy uses both direct and indirect actions and can include media campaigns, public speaking and commissioning and publishing research with the intention of influencing policy, resource allocation and decision making within political and social systems. Some of the different forms of advocacy include the following:

- Health advocacy supports and promotes health care rights as well as enhances community health and policy initiatives, for example, the availability, safety and quality of care. Brown et al. (2004) contrast health activism with health advocacy because the latter focuses on education and relies on expert knowledge rather than inserting lay knowledge into expert systems.

Activist-oriented groups, in contrast, tend to engage in direct actions, and challenge and insist on democratic participation in knowledge production.

- Media advocacy is the strategic use of the mass media as a resource to advance a social or public policy initiative (discussed in Chapter 6).
- Collective or mass advocacy occurs when groups and organisations campaign on issues that are important to their members and who then speak out for themselves or influence what others say in the campaign, for example, through protests (Loue et al., 2003).
- Peer advocacy is a similar concept of 'one-to-one' support in which a person agrees to act on the behalf of another and may belong to a support group, for example, volunteers who are recruited to act on behalf of service users at a citizens' advice centre.
- Self-advocacy occurs when individuals or groups share the same concerns or act on their own behalf.
- Legal advocacy occurs when a legally qualified person is employed to act on the behalf of others as an advocate, solicitor or barrister (Smithies and Webster, 1998).

In practice, the different forms of advocacy overlap, for example, self-advocacy groups can play an important role for supporting peer advocacy and collective advocacy can support the efforts of self-advocacy groups. Patient advocacy groups allow people to represent others and to speak out for their rights as patients (and as human beings). The example in Box 7.2 below is of a patient advocacy group that was supported by a health service employer.

Box 7.2   Patient advocacy groups

A hospital in the UK asked patients to pass on comments to staff or to make formal complaints, but there was no way of bringing together patient comments to effect improvement. The Patient Involvement Action Group (PIAG) was later established by the hospital to allow patients to voice their comments and concerns, anonymously if they wished, and have feedback about actions taken. Patients and their carers were given PIAG comment forms which could be returned to a member of staff or placed in a collection box. Once a month all of the comments, both positive and negative, were reviewed by the PIAG and action was decided upon at an appropriate level, or a report given about action already taken. The results of each action were posted on display boards in the wards to inform the patients and their carers of the actions taken. These included:

- Side rooms for infection control had curtains fitted to act as a screening door to prevent staff from walking straight into the room when a patient is carrying out personal functions.
- Frosted glass in some rooms, which the patients felt had made them feel like prison cells, was replaced with clear glass and blinds.

- Wards which suffered from solar glare received vertical blinds to improve conditions.
- Shelves were put up in bathrooms for cosmetics, sponge bags etc. to help patients to manage their own care.

Each ward was asked to nominate representatives of whom one would be available to attend each monthly PIAG meeting. The number of formal complaints decreased to less than 20 per cent of the previous level as patients gained confidence that their comments would be acted upon and that the ward environment had improved (Improvement Network, 2011).

Leadership qualities for activism

Through different typologies of leadership the personality of a leader occurs as a distinctly powerful individual, particularly in relation to attributes such as being charismatic, visionary, passionate, reflective, and politically savvy. Alternatively, typologies of competency, the ways in which a leader puts into practice traits in order to influence other people, place an emphasis on motivating, inspiring, collaborating, communicating, and empowering. Typologies, whether of characteristics, competencies, situational variables or styles, share the notion that leadership is divisible into observable components. The leadership relationship with other members of the group is especially important and the leader is not in isolation but is in an interaction with his/her followers. Good leaders are aware of the hard working efforts of the members of the activist organisation who, behind the scenes, strive tirelessly doing day-to-day and often mundane activities. Activist groups are often made up of volunteers and low-paid staff who can lose their motivation or become burnt out from constant struggle and slow progress. Good communication and self-reflection skills are also key elements and leaders have to be creative and be able to adapt to challenges of rapid change (Frusciante, 2007).

Leadership clearly plays an important role in health activism. Leaders act as figureheads, spokespeople, role models, strategists, visionaries and theorists. Ron Eyerman, a sociologist, and Andrew Jamison, an academic interested in social and political policy (1991), argue that activist leaders can change societal values and norms towards health issues. Leaders can also be the origin of new knowledge as intellectuals within the movement to reinterpret its vision and ideas. In turn, this can help to set new problems for society to solve and advance new values for ethical identification by individuals. The role of people in social movements is viewed as those that lead and those that are led. The leaders often occupy the 'space' created for them temporarily before they seek legitimacy elsewhere, for example, in academia, media and government. They establish their new identities and thus act as a vehicle through which movement knowledge can be dispersed socially. In this way leaders create movements and movements create leaders in processes within society to challenge conventional knowledge and wisdom. As the movements create new knowledge and leaders both become absorbed and institutionalised by society, they can create a bridge between new knowledge challenges and the established knowledge constructions. In this way, the legitimisation of the discourse on health has been influenced through the absorption of movement leaders either into, or their direct influence upon, the government, the academic and the private sector. This has been the case of the main themes, for example, of the environmentalists and the Campaign for Nuclear Disarmament.

Activist leaders are important both externally and internally. To the wider public, they are symbols of social concern. Inside movements, charismatic leaders can attract and retain members and hold a group together (Martin, 2007). Some social movements have used a model of promoting the vision and personal leadership of one charismatic individual. The leader may be effective but this keeps the potential leadership small and leaves the movement vulnerable. Once such charismatic leaders have gone, the vision is not continued and internal conflict means that the movement loses its impetus. Mechanisms must exist to ensure the continuity of vision even after charismatic leaders have left. A solution to the problem is selecting a mix of different types of leaders or else making a conscious commitment to sharing power and an opposition to formal hierarchy. Such groups might adopt consensus decision making and encourage everyone to develop a range of skills and play a variety of roles in the organisation. Leadership still exists in such groups, but it is leadership based on contributions and respect, not formal roles (Martin, 2007; Laverack, 2004).

Leadership skills

Activist leaders need a range of skills including:

- the sharing of power and institutionalising internal democracy within movements;
- a style of leadership which encourages and supports the ideas and planning efforts of others, using democratic decision making processes and the sharing of information;
- the ability to boost the confidence of participants and develop in them a belief that they can succeed;
- the ability to promote teamwork and to motivate those around them;
- conflict resolution, advocacy and the ability to connect to other leaders and organizations to gain resources and establish partnerships. (Kumpfer et al., 1993)

Exceptional individuals who have a shared commitment to public involvement are also important to motivate others and to develop partnerships. In one organisation, local people were drawn into the process of participation and with increased confidence and capacity became powerful advocates in their own community. A proper balance between leadership and lay people was seen as essential because conflict was found to occur when there was a lack of clarity of who had decision making influence (Anderson et al., 2006).

Box 7.3   Leadership and the abandonment of female genital cutting

Female genital cutting (FGC), also called female genital mutilation, comprises all procedures involving partial or total removal of the external female genitalia or other injury to the female genital organs whether for cultural, religious or non-therapeutic reasons. Most women and girls affected by the practice of FGC live in 28 African countries although it also occurs in Asia, the Middle East and in some developed countries. It is estimated that at least 100 million women are affected by FGC worldwide (World Health Organization, 2000). FGC can have a negative impact on the health of women and girls and may increase their vulnerability to infection from sexually transmitted infections. Early complications include haemorrhage, urinary tract infections, septicaemia, rupture of the bladder and tetanus. Later complications include infertility, genital ulcers, scar tissue and genital sores (Dorkenoo, 1996). For example, in one study in Somalia, it was found that 100 per cent of women had been circumcised and that infection was reported in 60 per cent and haemorrhage in 20 per cent of cases (Bayoudh et al., 1995). Molly Melching is the founder and Executive Director of Tostan, a Senegalese based non-government organisation. Melching recognised that the Senegalese themselves, and not outsiders, must be the ones to carry forward the social transformation for the abandonment of female genital cutting. Her decision was motivated by the understanding that these traditional practices are harmful to the health of girls and women, and therefore, violations of their human rights and not in accordance with their religious and cultural values (Reaves, 2007). This understanding was a cornerstone of the Tostan programme, driven by her inspirational leadership. Melching has been a relentless advocate and lobbyist for the causes of the abandonment of FGC, forced and child marriage and human rights. Melching's leadership and the leadership role of local women at the village level have been an important strategy in the success of the Tostan programme.

Leaders as managers

Leaders do not necessarily have the skills to motivate and organise people and may lack the experience needed in their role as a manager. Good leadership involves both personal and organisational qualities. Effective activist leaders certainly have charisma but in order to be effective they must also have characteristics such as a decision making style, networking and political efficacy. Activist movements need leaders that take responsibility for getting things done, dealing with conflict and providing a clear direction. Simply put, an effective activist leader must also be a good manager. The manager is an organiser, the person who decides what needs to be done and then gets other people to do it. To achieve this, the manager can follow a sequential set of stages:

1. Objective setting: an activist organisation may express its aim as a 'mission statement', within which its objectives are clearly defined targets of proposed change over a specific period of time. The objectives are measurable and the term SMART (specific, measurable, achievable, relevant and time bound) can be used to define the criteria for a good objective.

2. Strategic planning: activists can employ a variety of best practice strategies to help achieve the objectives of their organisation. Best practices represent the growing body of knowledge about services and strategies which have been evaluated and accepted as being effective. They are sets of processes and activities that are consistent with activist values, theories, and evidence, that are most likely to achieve the desired goals in any given situation. An important part of the planning process is formally defining roles and responsibilities for the different people within the organisation through, for example, job descriptions. This enhances the role of the manager through delegation, the passing on of responsibility to others, and supervision to keep a track of the activities that have been assigned to them as well as assisting them to deal with any difficulties that may have arisen.

3. The control of the use of resources: to effectively meet the objectives, it is necessary for the manager to analyse and organise the available resources, including skilled people in the organisation, knowledge, experience, finance, materials, equipment and time. What the activist movement can achieve depends on the resources at its disposal and therefore resource mobilisation is an important stage in the growth of an organisation. The ability of the movement to mobilise resources from within and to negotiate resources is itself an indication of a high degree of skill and organisation. Resources may be internal, those raised by or already within the organisation, or external, those brought into the organisation by its members or by a fund raising strategy.

4. To motivate, develop and train people at all levels to fulfil the objectives and to adapt to changing circumstances: change can be a threatening process but new ideas and innovations, that may be necessary for the growth or survival of the organisation, are more likely to be accepted if they come from within the organisation rather than from an outside source. Autocratic management techniques in activist organisations can create a lack of trust between the leadership and the members of the organisation. The involvement of the members of the organisation is therefore an essential part of introducing and adapting to change (Hubley and Copeman, 2008).

The leadership and management of activist movements is an iterative process in which people learn by doing, reflecting on the outcomes, learning from mistakes and by putting these lessons into practice. Some activist movements purposefully adopt a leaderless style, comprising fluid, shifting, autonomous groups and networks that are non-hierarchical. This makes the management of these organisations an especially difficult task but this role can be aided through 'tools' such as action plans, objective setting, strategic planning, training and from the experience gained through collaboration with others.

Effective leaders also manage time properly, foster a commitment at an early stage and maintain on-going involvement of all the members of the organisation in the cause. In particular, a steering group, task force or committee can be a useful way for the manager (who can act as the chairperson) to keep the direction of the organisation on track. The qualities of a successful steering committee are of people who are prepared to put time and skills into the process at strategic levels. The committee provides regular feedback to the members and an opportunity to reflect and act on the lessons learnt and is also prepared to follow-up on recommendations (Smithies and Webster, 1998).

Leaders as communicators

One-to-one communication is an important leadership skill because this allows a dialogue to develop between the leader and his/her followers. The dialogue is often based on a sharing of knowledge and experiences in a two-way communication that is necessary to help individuals to retain information better, to clarify personal issues and to develop skills. Verbal communication is probably the most common channel of relaying information although electronic media is increasingly important in international organisations. The relationship of leaders with their followers can be influenced by the level of control that they have through their choice of communication style. Listening is an important skill for good leadership and an active process as the leader needs to focus on what the individual is saying and if necessary help them to express his/her feelings or to give an opinion on an issue. When giving advice, the leader is exerting his/her expert and legitimate power to persuade others into actually accepting a subservient role relationship. The relationship grants the leader the right to prescribe advice while the other person accepts an obligation to comply with the advice. However, obtaining and giving feedback enables the leader to clarify what others want, that they have understood previous communication or retained skills. This may mean obtaining feedback based on specific information using closed questions that require short factual (yes/no) answers or based on an open form of questioning to provide fuller answers. Giving feedback is important for the achievement of effective communication and in particular positive feedback that reinforces the strengths of the knowledge or skills of others. The leader encourages others to share their concerns, feelings and opinions but still directs the discussion (Laverack, 2004). To facilitate this process, the leader can use their power-with in which power-over is deliberately used to increase other people's power-from-within, rather than to dominate or exploit them, discussed in Chapter 1.

Activists can also use well-developed tools to become more effective communicators to increase the critical awareness of others. Health literacy is essentially a repackaging of the relationship between education and empowerment (Nutbeam, 2000). What is new about health literacy is that education becomes more than just the transmission of information and is focused on skills development and confidence so as to help others to make informed decisions that will allow them to exert greater control on their lives (Renkert and Nutbeam, 2001). Awareness raising, education, communication and advocacy are all indirect strategies used by activist organisations. Health literacy as a 'tool' is dependent on the users having a level of basic literacy, that is, the ability to read and write in everyday life. Health literacy can be implemented at three levels:

- *Basic/functional literacy* – sufficient basic skills in reading and writing to be able to function effectively in everyday situations.
- *Communicative/interactive literacy* – more advanced cognitive and literacy skills which, together with social skills, can be used to actively participate in everyday activities, to extract information and derive meaning from different forms of communication, and to apply new information to changing circumstances.
- *Critical literacy* – more advanced cognitive skills which, together with social skills, can be applied to critically analyse information, and to use this information to exert greater control over life events and situations (Nutbeam, 2000).

However, whilst there is some evidence that aspects of health literacy do lead to better health outcomes, more research is needed in this area, both to develop quantitative and qualitative approaches to evaluating health literacy skills, and health literacy is worthwhile (Chinn, 2011).

In this chapter I have discussed the pivotal role that individual leaders can play in activist organisations and social movements. In Chapter 8, I discuss the role of collective or 'community' activism through the actions of civil society organisations and groups and the strategies that they can use to influence and apply leverage onto others.

8

Community activism

Working with communities

It is important for practitioners to think beyond the customary view of a community as a place where people live, for example, a neighbourhood, because these are often just an aggregate of non-connected people. Communities have both a social and a geographic characteristic and consist of heterogeneous individuals with dynamic relations that sometimes organise into groups to take action towards achieving shared goals.

As a working 'rule of thumb', a community will have the following characteristics:

1. a spatial dimension, that is, a place or locale;
2. non-spatial dimensions that involve people who otherwise make up heterogeneous and disparate groups;
3. social interactions that are dynamic and bind people into relationships;
4. the identification of shared needs and concerns. (Laverack, 2004: 46)

Within the geographic dimensions of 'community', multiple non-spatial communities exist and individuals may belong to several different 'interest' groups at the same time. Interest groups exist as a legitimate means by which individuals can find a 'voice' and are able to participate to pursue their interests and concerns. Interest groups can be organised around a variety of social activities or can address a local and shared concern, for example, poor public transport. The diversity of individuals and groups within a community can create problems with regard to the selection of representation by its members (Zakus and Lysack, 1998). Practitioners try to work with the 'legitimate' representatives of a community and to avoid the establishment of a dominant minority that can dictate community issues based only on their own concerns and not on those of the majority of the community. Practitioners need to carefully consider if the representatives of a community are in fact supported by its members and that they are not simply acting out of self-interest and self-gain.

The popularity of the internet has altered the traditional use of the concept of 'community'. With the advent of online communities, new types of computerised tools have been developed to aid user participation. Information and communication technology has removed the physical barriers to communication, for example, Usenet lets people participate in discussions that are classified by topic, each with many conversational threads from across the globe. Online communities, like traditional forms of community, consist of a diverse group of people who participate in virtual spaces with little social context and member identity. IKNOW and ReferralWEB, for example, encourage communication among community members by enabling participants to find others with whom they share interests and by providing a means to contact them. This facilitates social interactions in online communities and promotes communication by creating chat spaces, for example, Community Viewer and Chat Circle allows the participants to perceive the number of people present and the level of their activity, just as they would in a room in the offline world. Continuous linkage between voice and video channels is one way to give more social context to online communities, for example, Media Space, a computer-controlled voice and video network system, was developed to support awareness and informal interactions in business organisations. The video panel of Media Space allows users to see at a glance who is online and who is talking to whom. The internet has helped to promote 'global communities' and 'digital cities' by building arenas in which people can interact, share knowledge, experience, and mutual interests. However, online activity is still limited to those who are computer literate and have access to a computer and the internet, and this can exclude many people (Nomura and Ishida, 2003). The internet has been used to build community cohesiveness, as in the example from the town of Carlisle in Massachusetts in Box 8.1 below.

Box 8.1   The Carlisle Community Centre

Carlisle is situated within commuting distance of Boston, USA. The Carlisle Community Centre is an online community service whose goal is to understand what an online community service needs to do if it is to promote the ability of people to build trust and cohesiveness. On the Carlisle Community Centre website, members can conduct local school activities and local political activities anonymously. The Message Board is for simple postings, the Calendar is for events, the File Cabinet is for uploads, and the Links are for shared bookmarks. The Ballot Box lets a user put a question to a vote. The user provides a title, explanatory text, options to choose among, and the length of time that the ballot will be open for voting. Room members may vote only once and all ballots are secret with only the running tally of votes shown. Users may post comments on the ballot, thereby arguing their case for voting one way or another.

The design of the community centre web facility has several basic principles to make it more accessible:

- It should eliminate anonymity to ensure that people know with whom they are interacting when online.
- Access is provided to members only to the service and is not open to everyone on the web.

- The site offers a free online home for community groups, clubs and organisations that already operate within the town and existing members of these organisations can therefore meet online and interact with one another via the website.
- The site is accessible to as many Carlisle residents and employees as possible and therefore operates using multiple browsers, multiple versions, and multiple platforms.
- Unnecessary use of pictures and images are avoided as are features that might require a user to download a browser extension or add-in. (Patterson, 2011)

Working with civil society

The concept of civil society has had a revival of interest in recent years among researchers and activists and serves as an important point of entry for an analysis of many social, economic and political issues. Civil society includes people in both their social and professional contexts who share a common set of interests or concerns, including the totality of voluntary civic and social organisations and institutions, and which form the basis of a functioning society (Putnam, 1993). Civil society is much broader than the concept of a 'community' as it refers to a diversity of spaces, actors and institutional forms, varying in their degree of formality, autonomy and power. Civil societies are populated by organisations such as registered charities, development non-governmental organisations, community groups, women's organisations, faith-based organisations, professional associations, trade unions, self-help groups, social movements, business associations, activist and advocacy groups (London School of Economics, 2006). Whilst the interpretation of civil society is debatable, it does involve those institutions that are opposed to the state and that have values of community empowerment and emancipation. Civil society has a broad range of values and intentions, both positive and negative, and there is therefore an element of 'uncivil society' that acts as a counterweight to an overly optimistic vision of what civil society is or can achieve. Ironically, while many policymakers are concerned with the challenge of building civil society in transitional and developing countries, there is a feeling in many industrialised countries that civil society has been degraded and has become less a feature of everyday life. The concept of civil society has been criticised as a 'feel-good' factor that does not always account for conservative or repressive forces in the political arena (Lewis, 2003). However, the broad range of interests that make up civil society are often engaged in competition with one another to bring about social and political change in their favour. They function as discreet collections of people who instinctively create groups, organisations, communities and movements to address shared needs.

NIMBY, WIMBY, NIABY

'Not in my backyard' (NIMBY) and the term '**Nimbyism**' are used to describe the opposition by people, often local residents, to a proposal for a new development such as an industrial park, wind farm, landfill site, road, railway line or airport in their neighbourhood. NIMBY is also used more generally to describe people who advocate some proposal, for example, budget cuts and tax increases, but oppose implementing it in a way that would require any sacrifice on their part. NAMBI ('Not against my business or industry') is used as an equivalent to NIMBY by those opposing the business or industry in question. NAMBI is a term for any business interests that express concern with actions or policy that threaten their business, portraying its protest to be for the benefit of all. Such a labelling would occur, for example, when opposition expressed by a business involved in an urban development is challenged by activists, causing the businesses to protest and appeal for support. The term serves as a rhetorical counter to NIMBYs. Other terms such as 'Why in my backyard' (WIMBY) and 'Not in anyone's backyard' (NIABY) have also been used to express the opposition to certain developments as inappropriate anywhere in the world such as the building of a nuclear power plant (Hull, 1988).

The example of one NIMBY in Australia in relation to a toxic waste site is given in Box 8.2 below.

Box 8.2   NIMBYs in Australia

Werribee is a small town in Australia situated in an agricultural and market gardening area close to the city of Melbourne. In 1996, the Local Government Minister announced the siting of the toxic waste dump at Werribbee and Colonial Sugar Refining (CSR) were commissioned by the government to prepare an environmental effects statement with the intention of CSR becoming the implementing agent for the project. The announcement of the development of the dump was a sufficient emotional trigger for outraged residents to take personal action. Their focus was against the toxic waste dump which residents felt would be detrimental to the health and economy of the community. Individuals quickly organised themselves into a resident's action group called WRATD ('Werribee residents against toxic dump'). Local leaders soon emerged who would become instrumental in the development of this 'community of interest' and its rapid growth into a proficient organisation. Within a period of 18 months, the 'community of interest' had succeeded in establishing an effective campaign to raise public awareness and influence political decision makers. WRATD employed local experts who gave weight to a sophisticated approach of information dissemination, for example, a computerised operations centre and partnerships with the local university helped to broaden WRATD's expertise. The campaign was carried out in a positive and pervasive manner constantly working behind the scenes to bring about political and social change in favour of the Werribee residents. After an enormous show of strength by 15,000 residents, who demonstrated against the siting of the dump, and a petition of more than 100,000 signatures, the CSR abandoned the project (Strong, 1998 in Laverack, 2004: 56). Environmental researchers have shown that decisions about the location of hazardous waste sites have often been made in a top-down way, ignoring the concerns of local residents, including economic losses from falling house prices. The environmental justice movement specifically evolved in the USA to help empower poor communities to have a more active role in the decision making process regarding these types of issues (Cwikel, 2006).

Community-based action

As communities move toward social action, they become more concerned about, and ready to address, the broader determinants on the lives of their members. Understanding the way this works is important because at some stage communities are no longer willing to be passive participants but begin to take an active role in identifying and resolving their own concerns. The key point is that communities will want to address the broader underlying causes of their powerlessness and will want to become engaged politically. This provides opportunities for others to work with the community to enable them to take more control of their lives. A community that is action-orientated is able to organise and mobilise itself toward shared goals and through community-based organisations to take a role in shared decision making and problem solving (Braithwaite et al., 1994). The roots of community organisation are based on the work of Saul Alinsky (see Box 8.3) whose underlying philosophy was that people should be in control of their own lives. Organisation and development, linked to a collective struggle, became seen by those working with communities as a legitimate model to improve the health and lives of others through activities such as education, skills training and technical support.

Box 8.3   Saul Alinsky and social organisation

Saul Alinsky (1909–72) was an advocate for the poor and powerless and a community organiser who used his position to lever others to gain greater political influence throughout his career. Perhaps Saul Alinsky's most important work was his utilisation of techniques that attacked racial segregation, notably in Chicago. Alinsky's strategy was to motivate an African American community into an organisation that would be considered powerful. Alinsky taught that change occurred when one agitated to the point of conflict. Conflict produced the crucible in which organised power could be applied to provide the leverage for social change. Alinsky believed that people had to experience coming into their own sense of authority and apply power in social situations. He wrote in his book

(Continued)

(Continued)

Rules for Radicals (Alinsky, 1971) that change meant movement and that movement invariably created friction. To this end, Alinsky worked in creating a black community organisation that would push for better integration in Chicago. The result was the Temporary Woodlawn Organisation, later renamed The Woodlawn Organisation (TWO). One of the overriding issues in Woodlawn was the overcrowded, segregated schools. With Alinsky's proven grassroots strategies, his penchant for creating tension, and a flair for the dramatic, the TWO began social activism to force the issue of overcrowding and segregation into the public arena. The campaign began with 300 TWO supporters appearing at a board meeting. When the school board president refused to accommodate requests for some to testify, the supporters marched out. One of Alinsky's rules for change was that an enemy had to be created by which political power would become polarised. It was polarisation that created the lever for action. Alinsky believed that in social action one had to pick a target, focus on it (or freeze it), personalise it, and polarise it. This tactic is necessary because in a complex society, it is hard to attach blame to any one person. Alinsky's approach was structured, centralised, and required strong leadership but proved to be effective in levering political influence (English, 2007).

Community action therefore begins when people come together to address a local concern about which they are passionate. These groups are initially focused inwards on local issues for a relatively short period of time but later develop into longer term community-based organisations. To achieve their goals, they must still possess the necessary resources, capacity and have the preparedness to engage with outside agencies. They must undergo the same process of social and organisational development as, for example, groups addressing longer term issues such as improving democracy. Both are concerned with the distribution of power and both have the aim of bringing about social and political change to support their cause. The first example is about the struggle for power-over resources and decisions regarding local concerns. The second is about the struggle for power-over resources and decisions in regard to governance at a broader national level. Both communities reach a state of self-determination and are focused on achieving goals through their own actions.

Whether or not the community goes on to achieve its purpose will depend on a number of different characteristics that define the functional and organisational aspects of success (Jones and Laverack, 2003) that include:

- having a membership of elected representatives;
- the majority of its members meeting on a regular basis;
- having an agreed membership structure (chairperson, core members, etc.);
- members actively participating in the meetings;
- records being kept including of previous meetings and financial accounts;

- the ability to identify and resolve conflicts quickly; and
- the ability to identify the problems of and the resources available to the group.

However, community-based organisations have a limited resource base and a limited membership and this means that they often have little influence (Allsop et al., 2004). To have more influence they need to grow and develop to have an established structure, strong leadership, the ability to better organise their members, to mobilise resources and to gain the skills that are necessary to make the transition to form partnerships, coalitions and alliances (discussed in Chapter 9). The focus must be outwards to the environment that creates their needs in the first place, or offers the means and opportunities to resolving them. Once the community has become more critically aware and conscious of the underlying causes of its powerlessness, it can then take the necessary steps to engage politically and to develop actions to redress the situation to gain more power.

Pressure groups

Pressure groups are commonly formed on the basis of the interests of their members such as professional organisations and trade unions or are based on a particular cause such as animal welfare, environmental and human rights and a variety of political causes. The common aim of these groups is to change the opinions and attitudes of society and to influence the policy-making process, but not to govern (Young and Everitt, 2004). This description can also apply to advocacy groups and interest groups but differs from social movements which are able to be representative of an ideology of greater equity, with deeper and broader social networks, as much as being the champion of a specific cause.

There is an important distinction to be made between pressure groups that are supported by an outside agent such as a health service employer, and those that are independent and are formed by its members, for the benefit of its members. The following example in Box 8.4 below describes how women affected by breast cancer formed their own pressure group to act on behalf of other women and to influence government policy in regard to gaining better access to Herceptin®, a drug used to treat the disease.

Box 8.4   The pressure group for Herceptin®

Herceptin® is in a group of cancer drugs called monoclonal antibodies. It works by interfering with the way breast cancer cells divide and grow when a protein that naturally occurs in the body, known as human epidermal growth factor, attaches itself to another protein, known as HER2. Herceptin® blocks this process by attaching itself to the HER2 protein so that the epidermal

(Continued)

(Continued)

growth factor cannot reach the breast cancer cells. This stops the cells from dividing and growing. Only about one in five women with breast cancer have tumours that are sensitive to Herceptin®. Women's groups campaigned for National Health Service Trusts in the UK to fund the use of Herceptin® more widely to treat breast cancer. The minimum cost to pay for the treatment is well beyond the means of most women who have breast cancer. The high cost of Herceptin® owes partly to the expense of research leading to its development, but also to the extension of intellectual property rights under international trade treaties that prevents the manufacture of cheaper 'generic' equivalents. However, the trusts refused to fund the drug until it was licensed for use in the early stages of the condition because of safety concerns and the absence of a product licence for the drug's use. The trusts indicated that they would wait for a published decision from the National Institute of Health and Clinical Excellence (NICE). This decision outraged many women who established local groups to organise and mobilise themselves to try and bring about a change in the decision made by local trusts. The pressure groups consisting of ordinary mothers and housewives organised actions such as local demonstrations outside hospitals, petitions, sit-in protests and wrote to their Member of Parliament. At a national level, the women established a website to support others and embarked on an aggressive publicity campaign against the government. As a direct result of the pressure group, the NICE was put under pressure to make a quick decision on the use of Herceptin®. Eventually, the success of a high profile court case ensured that Herceptin® was approved for use on the National Health Service. This was largely because of the determined action of women that soon developed at the national level in order to have a wider influence on the distribution of Herceptin® to others (Boseley, 2006).

Another form of a pressure group are 'health consumer groups': a voluntary organisation that promotes and represents the interests of the users or carers of health services, usually formed at a national level (Allsop et al., 2004). These groups cover a range of health conditions including heart disease, mental health and maternal and child health. Health consumer groups are mostly charitable organisations and are focused on one particular policy issue choosing to use tactics such as sharing information, providing support services for its members, lobbying and raising awareness. Online resources to support the actions of these pressure groups, such as the Patient UK website (Patient UK, 2012), provide people with evidence-based information about health and disease. The Patient UK website, for example, provides links to more than 1,800 patient support groups covering a range of conditions as well as forums through which people can support each other and can come together to create support and pressure groups on health related issues.

The collective action among mental health service users in Nottingham in England, for example, developed into a national advisory network and grew out of the meetings held by patients in hospital wards. Whilst involved in the personal development of its members, the main aim of the group was to have an influence on shaping mental health policy and services (Barnes, 2002) and not radical reform. Mental health action groups are often unified through a history of resistance against a dominant and unresponsive medical profession which gives rise to feelings of an injustice as people living with mental illness struggle to gain more respect, dignity and autonomy. The risk is that pressure groups simply become actors in a process that actually enhances the legitimacy of government policy or corporate interests as they pursue their own broader agenda. This is because pressure groups usually have little influence and resources even if they are able to form some kind of an alliance or partnership with others that share their concerns (Allsop et al., 2004).

Mad Pride is a mass movement and international network of mental health services, users, and their allies who identify themselves as being psychiatric survivors, consumers and ex-patients. The movement started in response to local community prejudices towards people with a psychiatric history living in boarding homes in the Parkdale area of Toronto. In the 1990s, similar protests and demonstrations were being organised as Mad Pride in England, Australia, South Africa and the USA. Mad Pride activists seek to reclaim terms such as 'mad', 'nutter' and 'psycho' from misuse, for example, in the newspapers. Mad Pride activists have also used mass media campaigns to re-educate the general public on the causes of mental disorders, the experiences of those using the mental health system and suicide. Mad Pride celebrates the creativity, strength and resilience of the human spirit. It provides an opportunity to empower psychiatric survivors and raise public consciousness about human rights through various actions such as art, street theatre, music, poetry, protests and vigils. For example, the 'bed push' protests aim to raise awareness about the poor levels of choice of treatments and the widespread use of force in psychiatric hospitals around the world (MADD, 2012). Since 1999 MindFreedom has promoted Mad Pride events internationally and has established a Mad Pride International Coordinating Committee to launch Mad Pride around the world. MindFreedom International (MFI) is an international coalition of over one hundred community groups and thousands of individual members. It was founded in 1990 to advocate against forced medication, medical restraints and involuntary electroconvulsive therapy. Its stated mission is to protect the rights of people who have been labelled with psychiatric disorders. MindFreedom International is rooted in the psychiatric survivors' movement which arose out of the civil rights movements of the late 1960s and early 1970s based on the personal histories of psychiatric abuse experienced by some ex-patients. MFI supports mental health networks and organises activist campaigns in support of human rights in psychiatry and against forced drugging, solitary confinement, restraints, involuntary commitment and electroshock treatment. For example, in 2003 eight MFI members went on hunger strike to publicise a series of challenges which they sustained for more than one month thus forcing authorities to enter into a debate about the issues (MindFreedom, 2012).

Strategies for community-based actions

Ordinary people most often use conventional tactics to try to influence policy such as signing a petition, sending letters, emails or texts to a politician, delivering promotional material house to house, the boycotting of specific products or through democratic participation such as voting. People resort to more direct tactics when they feel that these tactics are not effective and then use, for example, protests and legal action. When these tactics also do not work, to legitimately gain access to resources and decision making they may resort to unconventional, direct and even violent strategies, for example, strikes, riots or mass boycotting such as the refusal to pay taxes. Strategies for community-based actions are discussed under two main headings: the disruption at, or of, a specific target, for example, mass demonstrations or staged events, and; raising the awareness of, or influencing, a specific target, for example, lobbying and leverage.

Disruption at, or of, a specific target

A general tactic and probably the most widely used in health activism is disruption through some form of coordinated mass action, often involving the occupation of property or space, for a relatively short period. Such action can be symbolic but also aims to cost other people, companies or organisations time and money, bad publicity, raise awareness and force a quick change in circumstances. Causing a disruption is seen as an end in itself, for example, stopping work on a building site or stopping the day-to-day running of a hospital. Activists undertaking disruptive tactics often use props and symbols as a way of mediating their message. Activists will climb buildings and drop banners, wear costumes and do other stunts to attract media attention, as shown in Box 8.5 below regarding the pressure group Fathers 4 Justice.

Box 8.5   Fathers 4 Justice

The aim of the Fathers 4 Justice (or F4J) pressure group is to champion the cause of equal parenting, family law reform and equal contact for divorced parents with children. F4J began as a fathers' rights pressure group in the UK and soon became prominent and frequently discussed in the media following a series of high-visibility stunts with the protesters often dressed as comic book superheroes and frequently climbing public buildings, bridges and monuments. Stunts have also included supporters storming courts dressed in Father Christmas outfits and one group member climbing onto Buckingham Palace (the official residence of the British monarch) dressed as a superhero. F4J was temporarily disbanded in January 2006, following allegations of a plot by members to kidnap the youngest son of the prime minister but soon reformed and protested during a live broadcast of a popular television show (Fathers4Justice, 2012).

Protest camps are another form of disruption, for example, the camps at St Paul's cathedral in London in 2011 to protest about the global economy. Activists also squat in a specific area to force a period of stalemate where the owners of the land or property must take them to court to legally win the right to evict. Activists will generally use a range of further tactics to ensure that they are not easily removed such as digging tunnels, establishing tree houses or setting up tents and makeshift shelters. The aim is not necessarily to defeat the opposition, rather to slow them down, cost them a large amount of money, win public support, and get the bigger picture onto the public and policy agenda (Plows, 2007).

'Phantom cell' structures are small, independent groups but also include individuals (solo cells), that challenge government policy. While it lacks a central command the simplicity of the strategy means that this type of leaderless resistance has been employed by a wide range of movements including animal liberation and radical environmental movements and anti-abortion activists. The basic characteristic of the structure is that there is no explicit communication between cells which are otherwise acting toward the same goals. Members of one cell usually have little or no specific information on who else is agitating on behalf of their cause. The cells are not susceptible to informants as there is neither a central command, nor links between the cells that may be infiltrated, and it is therefore more difficult for authorities to stop the development of such a leaderless resistance movement. Phantom cells are often based on resistance by violent means but the same structure can be used for non-violent actions such as distributing propaganda materials, using the internet to create boycotts, crop trashing and other high profile and one-off media events. Affinity groups are a variation of phantom cells and are small groups of activists who will mobilise each other during protests and demonstrations, allocate roles and look out for each other. Affinity groups will take part in many different actions but groups are most often formed at short notice. The Clamshell Alliance is an anti-nuclear alliance in New England, USA which spearheaded a movement against the Seabrook nuclear power plant during the 1970s. The Clamshell Alliance first used affinity groups of 3 to 15 persons to occupy the plant, to protest and hold vigils. The Alliance also integrated and developed consensus decision making and used guidelines and trainings to facilitate discipline in the affinity groups. Facilitators managed discussions and 'vibes-watchers' took care of the emotional needs of the participants and helped to motivate group energy. Spokespersons communicated the results of decisions made by the affinity groups to the coordinating committee of the Clamshell Alliance (ClamShell Alliance, 2012; Vinthagen, 2007).

Protests and demonstrations

Protests and demonstrations are an expression of objection, by words or by actions, to particular events, policies or situations. Protests can take many different forms ranging from individual statements to mass demonstrations.

Protesters organise as a way of publicly making their opinions heard in an attempt to influence public opinion or government policy. A protest can itself be the subject of a counter-protest by which counter-protesters demonstrate their support for the person, policy or action that is the subject of the original protest.

Some of the different forms of protest and demonstration used in activism include:

- Protest marches, demonstrations and rallies are historically a common form of non-violent action by groups of people often outside a government office or in a public place.
- Picketing, a form of protest in which people congregate outside a place of work or location where an event is taking place. Often, this is done in an attempt to dissuade others from going in (crossing the picket line), but it can also be done to draw public attention to a cause.
- Street protesters, characteristically, work alone, gravitating towards areas of high foot traffic, and employing handmade placards to maximise exposure and interaction with the public. A variation of the street protest can be critical bike rides, horse riding and vehicle movements.
- Lock-ons involve the locking of one or more activists to an object so that they are unable to be moved. There are many different types of lock-ons, from structures built in the ground or in trees, as part of a land occupation/ protest camp, locking onto a company's office doors, to the gates of military bases and to machinery, in order to cause as much disruption to proceedings as possible. The use of lock-ons can be risky for the activist, as they place themselves in the hands of others who are sanctioned to use reasonable force to remove them.
- Bulldozer diving or digger diving involves individuals and groups putting their bodies in the way of machinery. The usual setting for this is where land is under threat of construction or destruction with the aim to stop the machines from moving by trying to get on top of or underneath the machines as this tends to force them to stop (Plows, 2007).
- Die-ins are a form of protest where participants simulate being dead, for example, protesters simply lie down on the ground and pretend to be dead, sometimes covering themselves with signs or banners.
- A **protest song** is about perceived problems in society and challenges the status quo by championing a cause including labour strikes, civil rights, gay rights, communism and anarchism, peace and justice and women's rights. Protest songs can get across a particular emotional message, promote a unified challenge and in other ways use music for political purposes. Most types of music such as popular, jazz, blues, country, spirituals and gospel, rock and roll, rap and hip hop, have involved a protest theme or message, although folk music has been the more popular form. Protest songs are more pronounced at particular times and there was an upsurge in the 1960s coinciding with social and political upheavals, with the rise of the civil rights, student, anti-war and women's movements, serving to galvanise protests and to influence singer-songwriters (Cohen, 2007).

- Blogging and other forms of electronic networking have become effective tools to register protest and grievances to reach thousands of people.
- **Graffiti** is images or lettering scratched, scrawled, painted or marked in any manner on property to express underlying social and political messages. In particular, spray paint and marker pens have become the most commonly used graffiti materials. Graffiti is considered defacement and vandalism and is illegal.
- Other variations of protests include flag desecration, nude 'streaking', soap boxing, self-immolation (setting oneself on fire), sit-ins, 'tent cities', walk-outs, work to rule protests and book burning (Roberts, 2009).

Boycotts

A boycott is an act of voluntarily abstaining from using, buying, or dealing with a person, organisation, or product as an expression of protest, usually for political reasons (Metoyer, 2007). A boycott is normally considered a one-time event to address a specific issue although it may be for a longer period of time, or as part of an overall programme of activism. Boycotts can also be successfully coordinated through information and communication and technology to quickly gain support and to raise awareness using, for example, mass emailing and virtual 'sit-ins'.

Consumer boycotts are focused on long-term change of buying habits and are usually part of a larger strategy aiming for the reform of commodity markets, or government commitment to moral purchasing of products. Many animal rights advocates boycott clothes made of animal skins, such as leather shoes, and will not use products known to contain animal by-products (Glickman, 2009). Consumer boycotting was a hallmark tactic of activists in the 1960s and 1970s to try and punish corporations. By the 1990s, however, the trend was more towards developing standards and accrediting retail products. The theory was that an accredited product would be rewarded by consumers. For example, the Forest Stewardship Council (FSC), which was established by a broad coalition of non-profit groups, aimed to shift timber production to sources designated as more sustainable through accreditation and reduce the market share for products derived from the destruction of the world's great forests (Burton, 2007). Concerns have been raised that boycotting products manufactured through child labour, for example, may force children to turn to more dangerous sources of income. UNICEF has estimated that 50,000 children were dismissed from their garment industry jobs in Bangladesh following the introduction of the Child Labour Deterrence Act in the USA in the 1990s. Many children resorted to jobs such as stone-crushing, street hustling, and prostitution, jobs that are more hazardous and exploitative than garment production. The study suggests that boycotts may have long-term negative consequences that can actually harm rather than help the children involved (UNICEF, 2001).

The movement to promote breastfeeding provides another example of the use of boycotting as an activist strategy and is provided in Box 8.6 below.

Box 8.6   The breastfeeding movement

The breastfeeding movement emerged in response to the growing popularity of bottle-feeding. Around the turn of the twentieth century, companies had begun marketing bovine milk products as infant food. By the 1950s, bottle-feeding was more fashionable and considered to be superior to breastfeeding. In the developing world, early breastfeeding advocates argued that formula was expensive for poor families and had negative health consequences for babies. Meanwhile, in industrialised countries, white, middle-class women argued that breastfeeding was an important aspect of mothering. Since then, an internationally organised breastfeeding movement has formed to challenge multinational corporations, influence international policy, educate and support breastfeeding women throughout the world. In the 1960s, the formula industry embarked on an aggressive marketing campaign in the developing world. The breastfeeding movement gained momentum to organise a boycott of Nestlé products, a major manufacturer of infant milk formula, throughout the United States and which was soon emulated in Europe, Canada, New Zealand and Australia. The World Health Assembly adopted the International Code of Marketing Infant Formula in May 1981, the first international code for trans-national corporations. The code stated that companies should accurately label their products, minimise advertising, avoid distributing free samples to mothers and maintain high quality standards. Due to corporate lobbying, the code was passed as a recommendation (which is more difficult to enforce) rather than as a regulation. In response, various grassroots organisations soon formed the International Baby Food Action Network (IBFAN) to promote the code and monitor the formula industry's compliance. In 1984, the Nestlé boycott was suspended after the company agreed to abide by the code. After numerous warnings, the boycott was resumed again in 1988 and was extended to other formula companies due to grievous code violations. More recently, advocates have sought to increase respect for breastfeeding in public places, for example, in 2004, over two dozen 'lactivists' held a nurse-in at a Starbucks cafe in Maryland, USA after a mother was asked to breastfeed her child in the bathroom and not in the public area (Metoyer, 2007).

Raising the awareness of, or influencing, a specific target

Lobbying

Lobbying is the attempt to influence the official decisions of policymakers. More specifically, it is taken to refer to the direct and personal communication between a lobbyist and the policymaker. Criticised by some on the grounds that it affords undue influence over public policy to powerful and resourced interests at the expense of those groups that are already less favoured. Its defenders assert that lobbying is merely the manifestation by a group of its freedom of expression and a mechanism by which voters are able to communicate directly with elected representatives. The term probably originates from Members of Parliament in the UK who could be met by their constituents and others in the Central Lobby of the House of Commons in the nineteenth century. Lobbying is a feature of the policy-making process in every democratic system and lobbyists commonly describe themselves as forming a bridge between government and the governed, across which information can flow in order to ensure that policy decisions are better informed and that people can interact with policymakers more frequently. Policymakers also find it useful to be provided with information by lobbyists about the possible impact of a policy decision. Much lobbying involves a relatively straightforward supply of information, often in the interests of the group providing it. If a policymaker hears from the range of groups lobbying on an issue, they will be better informed about the issue and thus better able to reach a position on it. This should not imply, however, that lobbying is a wholly unrestricted activity. Professional lobbyists in some countries such as the USA must register with Congress and must provide information on their activities and expenditures. Most lobbying is directed at those policymakers who already favour a group's interests or at those who have not yet arrived at a firm view on an issue, rather than being aimed at persuading a policymaker to radically change his or her mind (McGrath, 2007a).

Grassroots lobbying

Grassroots lobbying is based on the idea that 'all politics is local', that the more constituents who write or call about an issue, the more likely their elected representatives are to pay attention to it. Grassroots campaigns, in which substantial numbers of voters contact their elected officials, can give politicians a signal as to how significant a policy decision may be. Grassroots lobbying campaigns in which politicians are contacted by large numbers of voters, expressing a strong desire for the politician to support or oppose a policy proposal, will also likely be highly influential. For example, in India, the People's Health Movement has conducted a number of people's tribunals where evidence of the lack of access to health care and its damaging effects have combined with lobbying and court actions to hold the government accountable to its domestic and international legal obligations to maintain health services (Peoples Health Movement, 2012). Crucial to the effectiveness of a grassroots lobbying effort, though, is not so much the number of constituent communications generated, but rather that all communications demonstrate the individual voter's genuine views and, as much as possible, relate those views to the constituent's situation. Grassroots campaigns often start when group supporters write, phone, fax, or email their elected officials to express a view about a given forthcoming policy decision. Another popular technique, known as a **Lobby Day**, involves a group's members converging on the office of their local political representative to meet them in an organised way to deliver their message. This signals a strong commitment to the issue. A variant of grassroots campaigns is referred to as 'grasstops' efforts, in which a group attempts to identify and activate a smaller number of particularly influential individuals. These may be the friends, former colleagues, or neighbours of the politician, or key local opinion formers such as business or religious leaders (McGrath, 2007b).

Political leverage

The notion of leverage is understood to mean that some individual actors bring varied experience, widespread contacts, and a longer track record than others and this additional input can be seen as advantageous to lever or gain greater influence. More specifically, leverage refers to the ability to influence people or events to get things done. Sometimes this may be through the application of funds that will attract further financial support from others or it may refer to the participation of others in achieving goals. In essence, the individual uses their assets, including their knowledge, expertise, past achievements and funds, as a 'lever' to help gain a greater political influence and to have a pivotal role both within their own context and in the broader arena. To achieve a pivotal role, it is not always necessary to reach a critical mass of people, but merely for individuals within the group to see themselves as part of the collective and to identify strategic pathways to influence health policymaking and resource allocation. Resources are seldom sufficient (even in higher income countries) and there are many competing interests. Consequently, the 'leveraging' that is carried out will have to include a political component to convince decision makers, who have control over resources, to invest in a particular issue and to listen to the knowledge, skills and expertise of local people (Rathgeber, 2009). Leverage is therefore used to raise the position of one person or group, while simultaneously lowering it for another person or group. It is particularly dominant in Western thinking where it is often used in association with economic or political accounts of power and is equated to wealth and income and subsequently authority and status. Leverage is a form of zero-sum power in which one can only possess x amount of power to the extent that someone else has the absence of an equivalent amount. My power-over you, plus your absence of that power, equals zero (thus the term, 'zero-sum'). I win and you lose. For you to gain power, you must seize it from me. If you can, you win and I lose. The decision making authority that goes with it is zero-sum and one has authority or social status by virtue of others not having it. There is a degree of flexibility here, however, since someone may have authority or status in one situation, relative to others, but not in another. At the same time there are dominant social forms of status or privilege, such as class, gender, education, ethnic background, age and even physical ability or sexual preference, which tend to structure power-over relations in social situations (Laverack, 2004). An example of this can be seen in the actions of the radical elements of social movements such as the environmentalists. To gain a seat in the corporate-government boardrooms where environmental policies were being formed, this movement engaged in 'direct action' campaigns that blocked effluent pipes and prevented commercial logging. Only when day-to-day life is sufficiently 'disrupted' by such protest are the conditions for negotiated partnerships created. Moreover, such disruptions may continue to be required to prevent elite groups from co-opting those with whom they negotiate, or turning their back on partnerships once the opposition has been placated. Thus, the environmental movement today, like other social movements, has groups that sit around the table in partnership with government and corporate leaders (Labonté, 1990) as well as more radical elements.

Leverage strategies differ according to circumstances, but the objective is to add to the level of influence that an organisation or group has by harnessing additional assets. The case study below, for example, shows how the highly competitive garment manufacturing industry can provide opportunities for leverage to stop the use of sweatshops.

Box 8.7   Sweatshops and political leverage

Over the past decade, the political anti-sweatshop movement has become a major advocacy network. Large garment corporations are vulnerable targets for anti-sweatshop activism. Their buyer-driven character forces them to survive in highly competitive markets. To make a profit, they must compete with other sellers over consumers looking for good-quality clothing at very affordable prices. To maintain and even improve their market shares and profit margins, they outsource their manufacturing to countries where labour is inexpensive and devote considerable resources to marketing. In the weakly regulated setting of outsourced garment manufacturing, worker welfare is jeopardised by the fast and flexible production needed to keep up with fashion. The anti-sweatshop movement has used the vulnerable and competitive image situation of the buyer-driven corporate world to push to improve garment workers' rights and social justice. Wanting profits and a good image among consumers, logo garment corporations are now forced to address sweatshop problems. The anti-sweatshop campaign has had some success, for example, in Indonesia, producers exporting foreign textiles and footwear increased wages 25 per cent faster than non-exporting producers (Micheletti and Stolle, 2007).

Campaigners against child labour in the UK in 2009 called on two leading high-street retailers to stop selling clothes made with cotton which may have been picked by children. Anti-slavery International and the Environmental Justice Foundation accused the high street clothing retailers Zara and its Swedish rival H&M of using cotton suppliers in Bangladesh employing child labour (Knudsen, 2007). These activist groups held protests outside the stores and lobbied politicians with a petition to create poor publicity for the retailers who did have to respond to the leverage applied by the groups and state that they would withdraw from these suppliers or that they were not aware of the circumstances under which the people had been employed.

In this chapter I have discussed how gaining political influence involves the creation of 'bridging pathways' as individuals move from personal action to the development of broader interest groups and community-based organisations and become increasingly involved with others. The 'bridge' is the link between personal and community activism. There are pivotal points on the 'bridging pathway' at the progressive levels of social mobilisation that enable people to move forward towards gaining greater control. These pivotal points also provide the opportunity for leverage by one group, community or organisation to gain more control, resources or influence over another. This is discussed in detail as a 'continuum of community empowerment' in Chapter 4 and requires organisations and the people who occupy them to increase their skills and awareness and to progress from an individual, often inward looking perspective, to a broader, collective perspective. Practitioners can act as a brokering agent to support people to strengthen their capacity and competencies, helping others to find a stronger voice and helping them to recognise that change can occur through joint action by progressing along the continuum. In Chapter 9, I take this discussion further to include the important role of networking and the relevance of partnerships, coalitions and alliances in health activism.

9

Networks and activism

Working with networks

A network is a structure of relationships linking social actors (Wasserman and Faust, 1994) that in turn are the building blocks of human experience, mapping the connections that individuals have to one another (Pescosolido, 1991). Social structures are not based therefore on categorisations such as age, gender or race but on the actual nature of the social contacts that individuals have and the impact on people's lives (White, 1992). There are basic principles that underlie a network approach and that can guide their development:

1. Network interactions influence beliefs and attitudes as well as behaviour, action, and outcomes.
2. Individuals both act and react to the social networks in their environment.
3. Structural elements (size, density, or types of relationships) of a network can change its level of influence. The content of the network, the transfers of material or non-material resources, provide an indication of the direction of that influence.
4. Networks are dynamic and so there may be changes in the structure as well as changes in content and membership.
5. Networks may support or be in conflict with one another, for example, family, peer, and official work-based networks may reinforce messages in regard to health or may contradict with the individual priorities of people.
6. Social interactions can integrate individuals into a network as well as to exclude and isolate them. (Marsden, 2000)

Networks set a context within groups, formal organisations, and institutions for those who work in or are served by them, which, in turn, affects what people do, how they feel, and what happens to them (Wright, 1997). While the home education of children has been practised in many countries, both out of necessity and out of choice, it is most popular and widespread in the USA. Recent estimates indicate that well over a million US children are being home schooled. Home schooling is a growing, heterogeneous network of organisations and individuals acting collectively in an effort to improve their children's lives. The decision to home school is motivated by four broad categories of concern: first, religious values, second, dissatisfaction with the public schools, third, academic and pedagogical concerns and fourth, family life. Families opting to home school are not a random cross-section of the United States. Home schooling families differ from the average American family in that they are more likely to be white, to be headed by a married, heterosexual couple, to have greater numbers of children, to have college-educated parents, and to have larger annual incomes. This is largely a social network of parents who provide about 90 per cent of the home instruction and are normally not in the paid labour force. Home educators work together and have formed networks to share teaching materials and ideas, taking their children on group field trips and engaging in other social activities. Home schooling parents have actively built a 'community' and the social interaction of its members helps to reinforce their decision to home educate (Collom, 2007) and therefore affects what they do and how they feel.

In a fundamental way, our health is a reflection of the quality of our relationships with one another and social networks offer many people the opportunity to strengthen the level of support and social capital in their lives. Social capital in the form of trust, social norms of reciprocity and cooperation resides in relationships, not individuals, and therefore in the social networks in which they participate. Active participation within social networks builds the trust and cohesiveness between individuals that are important to mobilise and create the resources necessary to support collective action. Putnam et al. (1993) have written widely on social capital and define it as the features of social organisation such as networks, trust, facilitated coordination and collaboration. Individuals invest in and use the resources embedded in social networks because they expect returns of some sort although resources are not equally available to all individuals and are differentially distributed across groups in society (Lin, 2000).

The history of the AIDS coalition to unleash power (ACT-UP) provides an interesting example of how an activist group was able to quickly develop through the use of networking to address an increasing health issue.

Box 9.1   The AIDS coalition to unleash power

ACT-UP was one of the first and most active pressure groups in regard to the AIDS epidemic that swept through the gay community in America. ACT-UP was formed in 1987 in New York by a group outraged at the government's mismanagement of the AIDS crisis. AIDS activism became an important component of the lives of people living with HIV/AIDS by helping them to identify and organise around issues that they felt were important. Membership in the activist group reflected a desire for social and personal changes in coping with the illness. Interacting with others through collective action can change people in a variety of ways including a greater sense of personal empowerment (Zimmerman and Rappaport, 1988). ACT-UP used motivational factors such as building relationships, social networking and participation to recruit more people. For both individuals and groups, ACT-UP provided a means to fight discrimination faced by AIDS sufferers from government agencies, social service providers, the medical establishment, the media and the public (Brashers et al., 2002). The primary mechanism of change for AIDS activists is intra-group and inter-group communication through networking involving active recruitment meetings, the mass media, encounters with allies and counter-movement groups. ACT-UP was especially effective at training its members in appropriate skills such as media relations, scientific debate and fund raising. Organisers formed a network of members who became recognised in HIV/AIDS communities as experts in the field. ACT-UP meetings focused on developing consensus among the members through debate followed by carrying out actions by interacting with and persuading outsiders to join the network. Because of the credibility they had established with many key decision makers, ACT-UP frequently met with government officials and industry leaders to debate changes in policy and this gave the organisation an unprecedented level of leverage and influence. The types of changes that ACT-UP had advocated included improving drug approval processes, changing immigration policies, and promoting education about safer sexual behaviour. One of ACT-UP's major victories was changing drug testing and approval processes in the USA including expanding access to clinical trial participation, decreasing reliance on placebo-controlled drug trials and accelerating the drug approval process (Brashers and Jackson, 1991). Because of ACT-UP's actions, community activists became a central part of the National Institute of Health's AIDS Clinical Trials Group, participating with researchers in the development of clinical trials and exercising voting rights on its committees. However, ACT-UP was also criticised for using inappropriate tactics, for example, protests against the Catholic Church in New York interrupted services and posters of a cardinal pictured beside a condom carried the message 'Know Your Scumbags' in protest of his public opposition to safer sex education (Brashers et al., 2002).

Networks and health

The ability of communities to empower themselves is in part dependent on their ability to build and maintain networks, including health networks. A health network is a structure of relationships, both personal and professional, through which individuals maintain and receive emotional support, resources, services and information for the improvement of their health and well-being (Walker et al., 1977). Social networks can be an indication of related behaviour, for example, the biological and behavioural traits associated with obesity appear to be spread through social ties. People who experience the weight gain of others in their social networks may then more readily accept weight gain in themselves. Moreover, social distance is more important than geographic distance within networks and there is an important role for a process involving the induction and person-to-person spread of obesity. Peer support interventions that allow for a modification of people's social networks are more successful than those that do not. Social networks can be used to also spread positive health behaviours because people's perceptions of their own risk of illness may depend on the people around them (Christakis and Fowler, 2007). One cohort study in California found that survival rates from heart attack improved with an increasing level of social support. People who were socially isolated had three-times the age adjusted mortality rate than those who participated in social networks (Berkman, 1986).

Individual involvement in a network can therefore have direct benefits to personal health because they:

- provide sources of information about health and health-related topics from other network members who have a high credibility;
- provide a source of emotional, practical and even financial support in times of difficultly from others in the network;
- provide an opportunity to apply pressure, influence and leverage through the participation of others and the collective action that this can create. (Hubley and Copeman, 2008)

Networks for patients

Networks for patients can be supported by an outside agency such as a health service employer, or may be independent and are formed by its members for the benefit of its members, both patients and health practitioners. Patient Concern (UK), for example, operates a network in collaboration with other active groups run by patients and volunteers on issues that matter to them, including:

- Protection for whistleblowers: to ensure that professionals are not afraid to complain when they see neglect, indifference and poor care. This requires a direct confidential whistleblower line and legislation to ensure that they do not suffer for raising legitimate concerns, for example, that individual careers are not damaged.
- Assisted suicide: advocating for a change in the law to allow physician-assisted suicide for the terminally ill.
- Save our beds: campaigning against the reduction of hospital beds.
- Complaints procedure: strengthening a complaints system for patients to have the right to an independent investigation of serious issues.
- Access to medical records: patients' uncensored access to their health records. (Patient Concern, 2012)

The Patients Association (UK) is a joint campaign with the *Nursing Standard* (a professional magazine) that aims to tackle poor care and the causes of poor care. It established the Network for Patients in 2009 with a group of over 30 charities to collaborate about common patient issues for better information and support. The most frequent complaints received by the Patients Association are poor communication; toileting; pain relief; nutrition and hydration. The Network for Patients is able to make a bigger impact than if each individual charity campaigned on their own. The Association addresses the shared concerns of its members including the 'duty to refer', for patients to be able to trust that their doctors are making sure they are getting access to the best treatment. Access to information is the best way to ensure this is happening and patient support groups are ideally placed to provide this service. Doctors cannot be expected to be experts in all fields and so it is important for them to be able to direct patients to other organisations which have the expertise. Doctors can then actively support patients in finding patient-support groups and networks that could help them with managing their condition (Patients Association, 2011).

Professional health networks

Networks have some features that are particularly relevant to professional groups such as public health, whose functions rely on the interactions between its members. Social relationships underpin network activity with a strong sense of professional identity and solidarity and offer individuals and organisations the opportunity to access complementary resources and expertise. However, networks require significant investment for their establishment and maintenance and may therefore absorb rather than unlock resources, at least in the short-term. Networks require a non-hierarchical management style which allows an interaction between its members and this is in contrast to the bureaucratic and hierarchical style of much of the public health sector. Networks are traditionally spontaneous and rely on voluntary support and engagement which also gives them their energy and creativity. As a part of the programme of UK National Health Service modernisation in 2005–6, public health networks (PHNs) were established to ensure that the limited specialist expertise and resources were more efficiently deployed to support the Primary Care Trusts (PCTs). Public health networks enable professionals to engage with a broader range of other professionals and agencies (Abbott and Killoran, 2005).

Examples from Scotland and Lancashire in the UK in Box 9.2 help to explain the function of the public health network.

Box 9.2   Public health networks

The Scottish Public Health Network is open to everyone in Scotland who has a professional interest and significant involvement in the wider health improvement agenda including staff from the National Health Service, local authorities and academia. The Scottish Public Health Network aims:

- to undertake prioritised work where there is a clearly identified need;
- to facilitate information exchange between public health practitioners, link with other networks and share learning;
- to create effective communication amongst professionals and the public and to allow the efficient coordination of public health activities. (ScotPHN, 2011)

The Lancashire Public Health Network covers the geographic area of Lancashire County Council, Blackpool, and Blackburn with Darwen Unitary Authorities. The

(Continued)

(Continued)

network is a partnership between the Lancashire Primary Care Trusts, Local Authorities, NHS Trusts, the voluntary sector and other organisations in the County and covers a population of over 1,445,100 people. The Lancashire Public Health Network aims to support the delivery of health improvement and the reduction of health inequalities across Lancashire by sharing learning and good practice, effectively using specialist skills and resources and by developing capability in the public health workforce (Lancashire Public Health Network, 2011).

Building partnerships, coalitions and alliances

Building partnerships, coalitions and alliances are crucial to empowerment and provide a pivotal point to collectively engage in activism because:

- they create shared values and collective goals;
- they can act as a 'common voice';
- they lead to the sharing and dissemination of information;
- they lead to easier communication;
- they can reduce feelings of isolation;
- they help with problem solving; and
- they help to reduce the duplication of efforts. (Kumpfer et al., 1993)

Partnerships, coalitions and alliances are seen to be a two-way process, one that is fully participatory and in which organisations do not merely consult with people but fully engage with them in decision making. The structure and function of partnerships, coalitions and alliances overlap but each has its own characteristics and these, with examples from practice, are provided next.

Partnerships

Partnerships demonstrate the ability of the community to develop relationships with different groups or organisations based on recognition of mutual interests and respect. Partnerships also demonstrate the ability to collaborate, cooperate and develop relationships that promote a heightened inter-dependency amongst its members. They may involve an exchange of services, pursuit of a joint venture based on a shared goal or an advocacy initiative to change policy. The purpose of a partnership is to allow an organisation to grow beyond local concerns and to take a stronger position on broader issues through networking and resource mobilisation. A key issue is that the members of the partnership are able to remain focused on the shared concern that brings them together, and not on the different individual needs in the partnership. But not all partnerships are equal. Barbara Gray (1989), a writer on inter-organisational collaboration, comments that 'weaker' partners must first develop their capacity before the conditions for an equitable partnership can occur. One of the key conditions for the development of a partnership is that no one party has the power to act unilaterally. Even in democratic systems some stakeholders can have almost monopoly power around certain issues and effective partnerships around these issues can only occur after successful political struggles and community mobilising efforts have given greater 'power' to less powerful stakeholders. Moving beyond conflict to partnerships, then, is only possible after less powerful groups have created their identity as legitimate stakeholders, their ability to mobilise resources and their ability to prevent the unilateral actions of more powerful stakeholders.

Partnerships can also be useful to help to build leadership and the 'Altogether Better' project, provided in Box 9.3 below, is an example of the success in establishing a partnership between government, private and public interests to support community 'champions'.

Box 9.3   The Altogether Better project

The Altogether Better project in the UK, launched in 2008, is a five-year regional-local programme designed to deliver innovative techniques to empower communities to improve their health and well-being. The programme focuses on community champions, facilitating a 'learning network' and building partnerships consisting of local communities, local government, universities and regional agencies. Altogether Better increases individual and community social capital, voluntary activities and wider civic participation and highlights the pathways to education, paid employment and enterprise. Altogether Better is made up of a diverse portfolio of 16 projects spread over 14 local strategic partnerships that aim to help individuals and communities to: eat more healthily; be more physically active; and improve their mental health. Exceptional people were identified as local champions by the project who helped to provide a focal point around which partnerships could later develop. Other participants were then drawn into the process and with increased confidence and capacity also became advocates for their own communities (Altogether Better, 2011).

Coalitions

The defining characteristic of a coalition is that, by uniting around an issue, different groups can enable their particular causes to be presented better as a broad issue rather than each group's narrow interests. Coalitions tend to be temporary arrangements that form to work around one specific issue by different organisations, even though they may oppose one another on other issues. As long as the end goal is shared, however, they can set aside their differences to work cooperatively. Coalitions also work because each member brings a particular resource, for example, knowledge, money or access to an influential person or organisation. The larger the coalition the more likely the goal is to be achieved because the members are better able to pool their resources in order to maximise the impact of their campaign. A coalition enables its members to argue more persuasively rather than as separate organisations. In other words, policymakers are more likely to listen favourably to the views of a coalition rather than similar views expressed by a number of smaller groups separately. Groups which do not commonly work together but nevertheless find it possible to cooperate on a particular issue in itself can suggest that the objective represents 'worthwhile' policy. Decision makers are able to communicate and negotiate efficiently with a coalition by minimising the confusion that can result from a number of groups, each lobbying individually on the same issue. A coalition can ensure that this level of negotiation and compromise is undertaken internally before policymakers are approached externally (McGrath, 2007b).

Once member organisations have been recruited into a coalition it becomes necessary to establish explicit guidelines regarding its organisation and management. Given that most coalitions are temporary arrangements focused on the achievement of limited goals, they have the potential to be relatively flexible. However, it remains crucial that a number of issues are resolved at an early stage. The coalition should ensure that there is a clear understanding of the joint objectives and ideology as this will help to reach an agreement, for example, about funding sources and the payment of members for services. All members must know which of them will be undertaking particular functions within the coalition, for example, who will coordinate the campaign and who says what, when and to whom. Some mechanisms for running and coordinating the campaign have to be negotiated, because the lack of financial support can be a reason for failure on the part of the people running the activities. The structure of a coalition can expose it to civil liability and it is therefore necessary for the members to agree upon a strategy and the key messages to be delivered, who will act as the spokesperson for the coalition for public announcements, media comment and submissions to government. This person can then have an independent legal identity, responsible for what is said with authority, rather than the coalition being liable (Fitzroy Legal Service, 2012; Rathgeber, 2009).

In building an effective health coalition the following eight steps have been used:

1. Decide if there is an advantage in creating a coalition.
2. Recruit suitable people.
3. Identify the aim and activities of the coalition.
4. Hold the first meeting.
5. Identify the necessary resources.
6. Identify the coalition structure.
7. Maintain regular meetings and energy of the participants.
8. Evaluate and provide feedback for further development. (Cohen et al., 1991)

Coalitions are useful only for as long as they stay focused on achieving a specific outcome. If each member needs to go back to their organisation for approval of decisions the process will inevitably become too time consuming and the coalition will cease to operate flexibly. The policy objective of the coalition should also be as focused as possible in order to minimise the chances of some members being pulled away as a result of concessions from policymakers (McGrath, 2007b). Successful coalitions are those that remain small and manageable and are able to both engage with community and involve its members in the development of future programmes.

Coalitions and the homeless

The meaning of the term 'homeless' gets alternatively applied to those who lack permanent housing, those who have inadequate housing, those staying in shelters and those sleeping on the streets (Mathieu, 2007). Homeless persons, as a group, are exposed to many social and environmental risk factors for health, and as a result are a serious public health concern. Even relatively short periods of homelessness expose individuals to severe deprivations, for example, hunger, a lack of adequate hygiene, physical assault, robbery, or rape (Bassuk et al., 1996). Those without housing often organise in temporary and tactical ways but the very challenges that make it difficult to be homeless (lack of stability, challenges to work, no reliable means of communication) pose significant barriers to social mobilisation. This is often left to advocacy organisations. The first coalitions for the homeless began forming in late 1970s and 1980s, working to put homelessness on the policy agenda and to lobby for emergency services and resources using, for example, street theatre and vigils to raise awareness. The formation of local homeless coalitions led to better organisation, for example, in the United States the founding of the National Coalition for the Homeless (Mathieu, 2007). Homeless coalitions work to tackle the root problems of homelessness, such as the lack of housing and to raise more resources for homeless people. The case study example of 'Street papers' below in Box 9.4 provides an insight into the effective work that coalitions can achieve by working with homeless people.

Box 9.4   Street papers and the homeless

In the late 1980s, street papers began appearing in major cities around the world. Street papers began as local initiatives, focusing on local issues and sold person to person on the streets. *The Big Issue* was launched in 1991 in response to the growing number of rough sleepers on the streets of London inspired by another newspaper called *Street News*, which was sold on the streets of New York. The philosophy behind *The Big Issue* was in helping homeless people to help themselves and to offer a legitimate alternative to begging. *The Big Issue* is now one of the UK's leading social businesses and continues to offer homeless and vulnerably housed people the opportunity to earn a legitimate income. The organisation is made up of two parts: a limited company which produces and distributes *The Big Issue* magazine, to a network of street vendors and a charity which addresses the issues that contribute to

(Continued)

(Continued)

homelessness. The organisation supports over 2,900 homeless and vulnerably housed people across the UK and the street paper is read by over 670,000 people every week in the UK. *The Big Issue* has helped to challenge and shape public perceptions of homelessness and has worked with over 10,000 individuals supporting them to address issues on health, housing, finances and employment. In the past decade, street papers have begun consciously seeking to effect change on a global scale by forming a coalition under the banner of the International Network of Street Papers (INSP). INSP has member papers located in 55 cities in 28 countries, their combined annual circulation exceeding 24 million copies and has begun initiating global anti-poverty campaigns via its Global Street News Service (Big Issue, 2012; Mathieu, 2007).

Alliances

A strategic health alliance is a relationship between two or more parties (individuals, groups, communities or organisations) to pursue a set of agreed upon goals while remaining independent organisations. The main purpose is to enable themselves, or that of others, to increase control over their lives and to improve health, going beyond health care (Jones et al., 2002). Members provide resources such as funding, equipment, knowledge, technology transfer, expertise or intellectual property. An alliance is a collaboration which aims for a synergy where each partner's benefits are greater than those from their individual efforts. To avoid facing unheated homes in the winter some communities have created alliances to be able to purchase heating oil at cheaper prices. These are called **community oil cooperatives** and the example below shows how such an alliance can be of a mutual benefit to all members.

Community oil cooperatives

In the UK some rural areas have created an alliance of between 5–9 villages to work as a cooperative to purchase heating oil in bulk from suppliers at more favourable prices. There are typically several buying cycles for heating oil in any one year and any residents who join the cooperative can participate in the scheme. At each buying cycle, community oil cooperative members are contacted in order to estimate their requirements as a fixed number of litres. An average household storage tank holds 2,000 litres and each member can order the whole amount or a smaller volume of oil. The cooperative is able to place orders of heating oil in excess of 200,000 litres and the total amount is used to negotiate the best price at that time from a number of different suppliers. Each cooperative has its own volunteer coordinator to collect orders and the details of the scheme are set out in guidelines. The contract remains between the resident and the chosen supplier. Therefore the resident has to pay the invoice according to the supplier's payment terms. Failure to do so may put the scheme at risk and would lead to the resident being excluded from the cooperative. The main advantages are that the residents can get heating oil at the same price per litre whether they purchase 500 or 2,000 litres. Even if they order the minimum amount of 500 litres they do not have to pay a penalty that is usually enforced by the supplier. This is a more equitable system and means that people do not have to risk running short of oil, especially in the winter because they have a low income, are unemployed or live on a pension. The disadvantage is that the coordinator does not know the discounted price before the cooperative order is placed with the supplier and so residents cannot budget exactly for how much they will have to pay per litre. However, the price is always cheaper than the normal retail order price from the supplier. The coordinator also does not know who the supplier will be in advance until the lowest order price is identified and placed. But once the supplier is chosen and the addresses of recipients are given by the coordinator to the supplier, a notice is posted on a website so that residents know when and from which supplier the heating oil will be delivered (Marton cum Grafton, 2012).

Building partnerships, coalitions and alliances inevitably leads to some level of compromise by one or all of the stakeholders engaged in the relationship. This means that over time the membership, organisational structure, purpose and ideology of the original relationship may have to change. However, this is not necessarily a negative development and can lead to the evolution of an even stronger and more effective collaboration. The case study in Box 9.5 below of the South African Treatment Action Campaign provides an example of how an organisation can create a stronger relationship with its partners.

Box 9.5   The South African Treatment Action Campaign

The South African Treatment Action Campaign (TAC) first mobilised around HIV treatment access in 1998, building from a number of self-help groups to become a national organisation with branches in all South African provinces and most major cities. It was started by two individuals who were angered by their countries' lack of response to the HIV pandemic and who realised that few self-advocacy groups existed for blacks, or brought both blacks and whites together around the issue of AIDS treatment. As TAC grew from a small group to a formal organisation, it included services to its members such as health care and education about HIV treatment. It also sought to broaden a base of local community activism and, through its educational and collective advocacy work, to increase the number of people working on its multiple strategies, some indirect, others direct, and still others of deliberate acts of civil disobedience

(Continued)

(Continued)

(Friedmann and Motiar, 2005). While TAC is only one of several popular social movements that arose in post-apartheid South Africa, it is credited with being the first to enjoy huge popular support (Endresen and van Kotze, 2005).

TAC is also credited with galvanising opposition to the court challenge brought by multinational drug firms against the South African government's attempts to import cheaper versions of antiretroviral treatments. It also lobbied its own government to move away from HIV-denialism to a belated (though still inadequate) Anti-Retroviral-Treatment roll-out. TAC advocated that health was a matter of human rights, a part of the South African Constitution. This argument was used by TAC in a successful court case that forced the government to dispense mother-to-child HIV transmission treatment. TAC created partnerships, alliances and coalitions with others involved in the labour unions and anti-poverty movements. In 2005, TAC commissioned an evaluation of its work (Boulle and Avafia, 2005) that found a shift from being a social movement with a campaign-driven focus and strong grass-roots alliances to a bureaucratic civil society organisation with specified projects and measureable outputs. This evolution has allowed TAC, unlike many groups in Africa, to continue attracting significant external funding (Friedmann and Motiar, 2005) and to expand its range of activist activities.

In this chapter I have discussed the role that networks, partnerships, alliances and coalitions play in promoting health and health activism. In Chapter 10 I bring together the key implications of using an activist approach discussed as key themes throughout the book and conclude what can work best and what kind of future roles activists can have in changing the way we design and deliver our public health programmes.

10

The future role of health activism

In this book I have defined activism as action on behalf of a cause, action that goes beyond what is conventional or routine, relative to actions used by others in society (Martin, 2007). Health activism involves a challenge to the existing order whenever it is perceived to lead to a social injustice or health inequality and uses a range of tactics that vary according to the function, structure and purpose of those trying to redress the imbalance of power that has created the situation in the first place. Historically, there are examples of how health activism has helped people to take more control of their lives but there are constraints on its use in a contemporary context leading to a shift away from its traditional form towards the more innovative use of information and communication technology. The aim of health activists, however, remains the same, past and present. To take action to redress inequalities in the distribution of power and resources that lead to negative influences on people's lives, based on their own identified and shared needs. This is especially important for people who are low on the social gradient and whose social conditions are shaped by having less economic or social protection from social injustice and inequality. Social injustice is today killing people on a grand scale caused by inequities in power, money and resources (Marmot et al., 2010). The perpetrators of social injustice are known to us and it is timely for empowerment and health activism to be used as a means to take action against them (Navarro, 2009). The perpetrators are the faceless multinational and national corporations, companies and capitalists to whom profits are the main priority. They are the bureaucrats, policymakers and governments that insist on an agenda of individualism and economic conservatism, to whom future cost-savings in health care services are the main priority. The role of health activism is to challenge the perpetrators of social injustice by using, if necessary, action that goes beyond the conventional. In this book I discuss the different tactics that can be used by health activists and have given case study examples of how these have worked in the past to influence the political drivers and perpetrators of social injustice.

Global economic conditions have given rise to many governments pursuing a tighter political and economic agenda. Public policies have been promoted that reduce social and economic structures, deregulate labour and financial markets, and stimulate commerce and investment (Navarro, 2009). Government policies are promoting economic conservatism, individualism and personal responsibility for one's own life and health. For everyday living conditions, this means that governments are cutting pay and jobs, freezing benefits and welfare payments and reducing opportunities for community empowerment, education and maintenance of the infrastructure (Nathanson and Hopper, 2010). This neo-liberal ideology is attractive to politicians because it (falsely) promises easily quantifiable and achievable results within a short time frame, and is relatively simple (Gangolli et al., 2005) and offers powerful financial incentives for savings in health care services, especially for people suffering from chronic diseases (Bernier, 2007). Governments are further reducing their responsibility by increasing market choice, transforming national health services into insurance-based health care systems, privatising medical care and by promoting a bio-medical model of health as individual behaviour change (Navarro, 2009). To counter-act these changes, we need a stronger political statement, one for radical societal change and a revolutionary call for action.

Health activism has been a successful strategy for small pressure groups, focusing on a specific, sometimes localised and often short-term issue. The chances of success are greatly improved if the issue has a simple policy or practice solution, for example, women's pressure groups in the UK successfully campaigned for more funding for the use of Herceptin® to treat breast cancer because the minimum cost to pay for the treatment was well beyond the means of the women with breast cancer (Boseley, 2006).

Activism has also had an important role to help social movements to carry out broader, long-term campaigns such as the birth-control movement for better choices for women in Chapter 7 (Daly, 2007) and the breastfeeding movement in Chapter 8 (Metoyer, 2007). Social movements that have been successful have employed a combination of tactics, have strong leadership, good media relations, a network of strategic alliances and sufficient, independent financial resources. For example, the South African Treatment Action Campaign (TAC) (discussed in Chapter 9) is credited with galvanising opposition to the court challenge brought by multinational drug companies against the South African government's attempts to import cheaper versions of antiretroviral treatments. TAC successfully employed direct tactics including civil disobedience, legal action, media advocacy and the leaking of government documents to force it to make antiretroviral drugs available through the public health system (Friedmann and Motiar, 2005).

In this the final chapter I discuss some of the challenges that activists face in influencing the perpetrators of social injustice such as individualism and an unsupportive political environment. I also discuss the future role of health activism in addressing health inequalities through a strategy of 'working together' with other stakeholders.

Individualism and health

Individualism is an ideology that holds people responsible for their own actions and the consequences that these may have. In ethical terms individualism refers to the ability of a person to make fully autonomous choices to take control of their lives and health (Tengland, 2007). Health is individualised by people who regard it as personal in nature and there can be a tendency to blame victims for their ill health, as people are responsible for the things, both good and bad, that happen to them. However, those defined as 'victims' may identify themselves with the term and feel that they do not have the right or do not possess the motivation to change their circumstances. The shift in politics in Westernised countries from ideologies of the left (social liberals, democrats, socialists and communists) toward the right (conservatives, capitalists, nationalists) have made individualism more influential in public health policy (Baum, 2008). Government health agendas typically promote individual healthy lifestyles to address issues based on scientific and epidemiological evidence, for example, the prevalence of obesity and heart disease in society. Government-funded programmes use motivational interventions that target the general population to adopt healthy lifestyles and to change their 'unhealthy' individual behaviours. These programmes typically increase awareness and develop personal skills to encourage exercise, eating a balanced and nutritious diet, not smoking and the moderate use of alcohol. A paradox is that targeting the behaviour of the majority who are at a low to medium risk, through top-down interventions, has little effect at the individual level. For example, reducing dietary fat consumption for the whole population would reduce coronary heart disease, but it is difficult to change the behaviour of the majority of people whose risk is only low to medium (Hunt and Emslie, 2001). It is also difficult to change the behaviour of people who are typically not captured by top-down interventions, such as ethnic minority groups, due to socio-cultural constraints. The modest success of individualistic strategies targeting a modification of 'unhealthy' lifestyles has mostly been with the educated and economically advantaged in society. For example, between 1998 and 2004, there was a 9 per cent decrease in smoking in the lowest quintile in Australia compared to a 35 per cent decrease in the highest quintile (Baum, 2007: 91). Likewise, between 2000 and 2005, top-down efforts in Saskatchewan, Canada, to increase physical activity resulted in 30 per cent people becoming more active but at the same time 14 per cent becoming less active. The change in physical activity had occurred in the higher socio-economic groups with little or no effect on the low socio-economic, adolescents, ethnic minorities or indigenous people (Saskatoon Regional Health Authority, 2005). As a consequence, public health may have had little effect in closing the gap between the 'healthy wealthy' at the top of the social gradient and low socio-economic groups further down. It may even, at least temporarily, have led to an increase in health inequalities (Baum, 2007).

Public health may not therefore be directly addressing peoples' health needs but neither is it listening to what people really want. The simple logic of individualism and victim blaming ignores the complex set of factors that make changing behaviour difficult and the social, economic and political circumstances in which decisions are taken. Peoples' behaviour is a reflection of the context in which they live. A person who is low in the social gradient may use their autonomous choice to smoke and to eat unhealthy foods because it helps them to reduce stress and gives them pleasure. It is no surprise then that top-down programmes focusing on specific 'unhealthy' behaviours largely fail to reach many people in society (Baum, 2007).

The framing of health as individualised creates an obstacle for activism. The personalisation of health provides a focus on the 'struggle', 'fight' or 'battle' against a disease or illness. The emphasis is on self-blame, personal responsibility and individual action. Individuals may be committed to change but this is only at the personal level and does not address the broader structural level. People who are passionate, even angry about, for example, climate change or the poor state of the global economy, are mobilised to protest about an issue that affects us all. But obesity and heart disease affect us individually, and the response is to deal with these issues at a personal level. The issue is not perceived as a threat to us all and this makes collective action difficult. However, there have been exceptions, for example, the collective action of the gay community in the 1980s to cope with the effects of HIV/AIDS. Such was the determination of this community that the extent of interaction was probably not seen before in regard to a health issue by both the medical profession and groups within civil society (Brashers et al., 2002). The spread of HIV was perceived as a threat by gay men to other gay men and this motivated many of them to act collectively.

Creating a supportive political environment for health activism

The account of Rudolf Virchow in Chapter 7 argues that all diseases have political as well as pathological causes. Health activism is political as its actions depend on, and have consequences for, the political context in which it occurs. Those in governance with decision making control can be supportive (democratic, liberal and egalitarian) or unsupportive (undemocratic, authoritarian and inegalitarian) towards health activists. Supportive political contexts provide numerous channels for the involvement of civil society, have multiple political parties, a free and fair electoral system and a 'free media'. There is a clear and constitutional separation of political parties, the legal system, corporate and church authorities and these include the UK, USA and many Western European countries (Baum, 2008). In a supportive political context, people are able to participate in a meaningful way but there are political circumstances that are even more likely to address social injustice and these include:

- the presence of 'left' political parties to influence government decision making;
- proportional representation electoral systems that increase the likelihood of such a presence;
- a historic state commitment to active labour policy, support for women's employment, adequate spending to support families, assistance for the unemployed and those with disabilities, provision of educational and recreational opportunities, and efforts to reduce social exclusion and promote democratic participation;
- high union density and effective labour powers to negotiate favourable wage and employment conditions; and
- the presence of strong civil society organisations with similar commitments. (Bryant, 2006)

Overall, it is a social democratic model that has been most committed to economic and social policies and supportive of public health and community action in developed countries (Navarro and Shi, 2001). The New Zealand Prostitutes Collective, for example, (discussed in Chapter 4) was able to work with the government in a democratic and liberal political environment, to take advantage of the timing of the national profile of HIV/AIDS as a key public health concern and to leverage its influence for the passing of legislation regarding the decriminalisation of prostitution.

Unsupportive political contexts have closed leadership, are authoritarian and are highly regimented, often with just one political party and no free and fair electoral or legal system. Examples of these types of political systems include the former eastern bloc, Middle Eastern countries and China (Baum, 2008). Under these circumstances, people must seize control through collective action, first at a localised level, and then through broader social and political change, making strategic decisions about what tactics they can use. Oppressive or hegemonic forms of governance, dominated by elite group interests, do not allow civil society organisations to function but neither can people rely upon support from the state. Community action is tightly controlled and people must therefore use the only significant resource they have, the capacity to cause trouble. The tactics used are unconventional and increasingly disruptive. The civil disobedience, public support and the reaction of the government become the basis for political influence. It is a risky option but one that historically has given rise to dramatic social and political change (Piven and Cloward, 1977); for example, the Arab Spring in North Africa (Abulof, 2011) and the Orange Revolution in Ukraine (Morozov, 2009) both used civil disobedience to successfully bring about political change in their countries.

The role of activism in addressing social injustice and health inequality

Action to address the political drivers that give rise to social injustice and health inequality requires that power and resources be redistributed by governments and corporations, from people at the top to those lower down the social gradient (Marmot et al., 2010). But how are these radical changes to come about? Will politicians and corporations willingly share their power and resources with marginalised, disenfranchised and minority groups in society (Nathanson and Hopper, 2010)? It would be naïve to expect this to happen. The development of government policy, for example, is complex and in reality is mostly undertaken internally, and in confidence, with minimal public engagement or practitioner and researcher involvement. Radical action is therefore sometimes necessary. Health activism is a direct expression of public discontent with government or corporate decision making. Those people most likely to be affected by government decisions, because they are low on the social gradient and have less economic or social protection from changes in, for example, taxation, benefit and welfare policies, have to challenge policy and legislative formulation or stop its approval. People can use conventional action to express their discontent by attending a planning meeting, voting, signing a petition or writing a letter to lobby someone in a decision making position. However, those who are low on the social gradient are often unsuccessful in using such an indirect strategy because they lack the resources and political leverage necessary to have an influence. People who can persuade others to make changes do so by using direct tactics that include a show of support, for example, through mass demonstrations. These actions are also symbolic, challenging government decisions and sending a message to politicians and policymakers about their grievances. The purpose is to shift political opinion about a particular decision, especially when it favours one group's interests or has not yet arrived at a firm view on an issue. However, if necessary people can also use stronger tactics to force others to change their mind through, for example, legal action and disruptive behaviour such as strikes.

Politicians are sensitive and react to the pressure applied by those activists who are able to play to the strengths of their position within a particular social, political and economic context. Between 2006 and 2010, for example, the New York City Food Movement (NYCfm) made progress in changing food policy, and the creation of new programmes and engagement of new voices influenced media coverage of food issues (discussed in Chapter 5). The NYCfm used a variety of tactics including open network meetings, websites, advocacy and information sharing and played a key role in the approval of the local initiatives to provide affordable food in inner city areas. The NYCfm was also able to seize the opportunity to have a lobbying influence in the passing of policies because politicians were divided about appropriate actions (Freudenberg et al., 2011).

Health activism is important because it can create the conditions for people to take control over their own lives when others cannot or will not act on their behalf. And people do have an obligation to challenge the perpetrators of social injustice and inequality because it is they that create the conditions that lead to their poor health and miserable lives.

The future role of health activism

In a rapidly changing technological environment, activism has evolved to take advantage of the availability of new ICT and applications such as SMS, Facebook and Twitter. This has enhanced the ability of health activists to communicate better, to organise, to mobilise, to lever funding and to access resources. The use of ICT has rapidly changed the way in which people are able to network and to present a 'face' for their cause with which the public can interact, for example, through a website. This means that there has been an increasingly important role for ICT to help reframe the debate at an international, national and local level. Online organisations are creating a new style of activism, often run by politically savvy, young entrepreneurs with a background in marketing, one that fully utilises the availability of ICT.

GetUp (GetUp!, 2012) is an independent, online advocacy organisation which aims to build a more progressive Australia by giving people the opportunity to get involved and hold politicians accountable on important issues. GetUp does not back any particular party and is a not-for-profit organisation that relies on small donations to fund its campaigns on problem gambling, same sex marriages and the rights of refugees and asylum seekers. The tactics that GetUp employs include information sharing, e-petitions to members of parliament, lobbying, media advocacy and networking. GetUp runs its campaigns from a website which is media friendly, providing easy access to information for journalists and taking targeted and strategic action to influence policymakers.

Dot-com activist organisations have several advantages over traditional forms of activism. For example, they are cheap and relatively easy to establish and can create a quick and international coverage of target audiences. They can include a number of issues rather than be focused on one and the technology that they use means they appeal to a young and energetic membership.

Avaaz is a global civil society organisation that promotes activism on issues such as climate change, human rights, corruption and poverty (Avaaz, 2012). The organisation operates in multiple languages, funding media campaigns, sending e-petitions, lobbying governments, organising 'offline' protests and media advocacy events. Avaaz's philosophy is that social movements in the past have had to build a constituency for each separate issue, year by year and country by country, in order to reach a scale that could make a difference. But by taking advantage of new technology, global civil society organisations, such as Avaaz, can be composed of issue-specific networks of national chapters, each with its own staff, budget, and decision making structure that can work on any issue of public concern in a flexible way. Avaaz's online community is polled every year to identify the most important issues to its members. Avaaz then sends email alerts to the online community in order for them to decide whether to get involved and if enough people participate, the campaign then begins to take momentum (Avaaz, 2012).

Working together for change

Activists that have worked with health practitioners to further their cause, engaging with leaders who are open to debate and to creating opportunities for dialogue, have managed to gain success. Professional bodies have used their 'expert power' to legitimise the concerns of others, for example, the support of the medical profession to the political lobby for the stricter legal regulation of boxing (Brayne et al., 1998) based on health grounds and for the pressure group Action on Smoking and Health to ban smoking in public places (ASH, 2012). Activists have also worked with health researchers to access evidence documenting problems and enumerating the benefits of policy proposals to support their cause. The public is open to rational discussion and activists are right to engage with practitioners and researchers to seek advice that is based on sound scientific evidence (Haynes et al., 2011). In fact, the combination of science and activism used by social reformers to change government policy is not a new idea and takes us back to the development of key public health legislation such as the 1833 Factories Act (Baggott, 2000) in the nineteenth century.

It is the combination of activism, a strong professional lobby and credible scientific evidence that has the best chance of influencing social and political change. Health activism can play an important role by helping to shape the debate and by pushing for change underpinned by rationality, research and action. This is a strategy of 'working together for change' using a combination of scientific evidence, professional support and activism, including social movements. Social movements are important because whilst they provide a substantial resource and participant base to support a cause, they also have the ability to maintain an ideology irrespective of membership, function and organisational structure. To do this, a movement must have 'deep social roots' and networks to maintain a momentum that research evidence, professional endorsement and public support alone could not achieve.

There is further evidence that a strategy of 'working together for change' has been successful, for example, in the use of seat belts in vehicles (Baum, 2008: 571) and for radical changes in surgical treatment for breast cancer (Lerner, 2001). Stakeholders with different levels of power and different skills can work together effectively to change public and political opinion. After the first AIDS case was reported in 1981 in America, the epidemic soon spread and the country found itself in the middle of an AIDS crisis. For the next decade, the public health services were stretched to deal with the increasing number of cases and for the prevention of the spread of the disease. The role between scientists and lay outsiders overlapped as the gay community mobilised itself to take more control to cope with the effects of the disease. Medical researchers, activists, policymakers and people affected by the disease worked together as a synergy motivated by the magnitude of the epidemic. The different groups sometimes fought against one another but as an alliance they worked in solidarity to try and understand more about HIV/AIDS. From the start of the AIDS epidemic there were calls for greater solidarity between affected groups and for better support from the public health services. Consequently, through their response and capacity to work together, by both activist and professional groups, public opinion shifted in support of those coping with the disease (Brashers et al., 2002).

'Working together for change' as a future role of health activism will depend therefore on its ability to do the following four things well:

1. To work in partnership with other stakeholders including researchers and health professionals to give it a better chance of success in regard to social and political action focused on specific policy change.
2. To adapt to new information and communication technologies that offer flexible and low cost alternatives to mobilise people, to recruit new members, to raise funds and to undertake activist tactics. These technologies are constantly developing innovative ways that activists can use to communicate, to network and to reframe the debate on relevant issues.
3. To work towards creating a supportive political environment for activism.
4. To challenge social injustice and health inequalities through collective action employing both conventional and unconventional tactics to achieve change.

In this book, I explain the foundations and strategies of health activism. I offer a role for health activism that will help others to address social injustice and inequality by gaining more control over their lives. Health agencies and the practitioners that they employ, professional organisations and researchers also have an important role to play in addressing these issues. What is clear is that if we do not challenge top-down programming, individualism, corporations and complacent governments, we will continue to have limited success in improving peoples' lives and health. The way forward for activists is not a revolutionary reorientation of the way they work but in an acceptance of activism as a legitimate approach in the way we deliver health programming. Health activism offers an alternative way forward at a time when innovative ideas are lacking in practice. The extent to which this happens will depend on our willingness to engage with activists and to work with them to address the causes of social injustice and health inequalities in society.

Glossary of terms

Activism Action on behalf of a cause, that goes beyond what is conventional or routine.

Advocacy People acting on behalf of themselves or on behalf of others to argue a position and to influence the outcome of decisions.

Affinity groups Small groups of activists who will mobilise each other during protests and demonstrations, allocate roles and look out for each other.

Alliance A relationship between two or more parties (individuals, groups, communities or organisations) to pursue a set of agreed upon goals while remaining independent organisations.

Boycott An act of voluntarily abstaining from using, buying, or dealing with a person, organisation, or product as an expression of protest, usually for political reasons.

Citizen journalism People playing a role in the process of collecting, reporting, analysing and disseminating news and information.

Coalition A temporary arrangement that is formed to work around one specific issue, often with another organisation.

Community-based ecological resistance movements Local movements devoted to the prevention of community life from environmentally harmful activities and the mobilisation of people in resistance to the issue.

Community oil cooperatives An alliance of communities to work as a cooperative to purchase heating oil in bulk from suppliers at more favourable prices.

Consumer boycotts Boycotts that are focused on long-term change of buying habits and are usually part of a larger strategy aiming for the reform of commodity markets, or government commitment to moral purchasing of products.

Corporate social responsibility Also called corporate conscience, corporate citizenship, social performance, or responsible business. A form of self-regulation integrated into a business plan or model.

Critical consciousness   The ability to understand the underlying causes of one's powerlessness by reflecting on the assumptions underlying our and others' ideas and actions.

Crop trashing   A tactic to destroy or damage field-scale trials for genetically modified crops and crop squats, protest camps in fields that are to be planted with a genetically modified crop.

Cyber-terrorism   The use of electronic communication technologies to undermine the security of the internet as a free social and political platform.

Digger diving   Individuals and groups putting their bodies in the way of machinery.

Empowerment   A process by which communities gain more control over the decisions and resources that influence their lives and health.

Environmentalism   An ideology regarding concerns for environmental conservation and improvement of the health of the environment.

Equity   A normative judgment of what is fair.

Graffiti   Images or lettering scratched, scrawled, painted or marked in any manner on property to express underlying social and political messages.

Grassroots lobbying   Based on the principle that 'all politics is local', that the more constituents who write or call about an issue, the more likely their elected representatives are to pay attention to it.

Grounded citizens' jury   An approach for local involvement in health decision making that can be used as a 'grounded' tool for activism in which local people are the agents in the development of policies directly affecting their lives.

Guerrilla television   The production of representations by activists of everyday reality to provide an 'insider's point of view' using home video cameras or community-based equipment.

Hacktivism   The use of computer networks as a means of protest to promote political ends through the non-violent use of illegal or legally available digital tools.

Hard power   Compliance through direct and coercive methods to compel others to do what you want them to do, whether they want to do it or not.

Health activism   In simple terms, health activism involves a challenge to the existing order whenever it is perceived to influence peoples' health negatively or has led to an injustice or an inequity.

Information and communication technology (ICT) A general term for the integration of telecommunications, computers, software and audio-visuals that enables users to create, access, store, transmit, and manipulate information.

Intactivists Genital integrity activists who oppose genital modifications, including genital mutilation and sexual reassignment surgery and are committed to the recognition of the right of all human beings to an intact body.

Internet activism (e-activism and cyberactivism) The use of electronic communication technologies such as email for unconventional activities to raise awareness, to quickly mobilise people or to evoke a reaction to an event.

Lay epidemiology A term to describe the processes by which people in their everyday life understand and interpret risks, including risks to their health and well-being.

Leverage Means that some individual actors bring varied experience, widespread contacts, and a longer track record than others and this additional input can be seen as advantageous to lever or gain greater influence.

Lobby Day Group members converge on the office of their local political representative to meet them in an organised way to deliver their message.

Lock-ons The locking of one or more activists to an object so that they are unable to be moved.

Media advocacy To influence the selection, framing and debate of specific (health) topics by using the mass media.

Moral suasion The act of trying to use moral principles to influence individuals and groups to change their practices, beliefs and actions.

Network A structure of relationships linking social actors.

Nimbyism The opposition by people, often local residents, to a proposal for a new development such as an industrial park, wind farm, landfill site, road, railway line or airport.

Partnerships Relationships with different groups or organisations based on recognition of overlapping or mutual interests and interpersonal and inter-organisational respect.

Photovoice A process by which people can identify, represent, and enhance their community through a specific photographic technique.

Phantom cells Small, independent groups, but also including individuals (solo cells), that challenge government policy.

Picketing   A form of protest in which people congregate outside a place of work or location where an event is taking place.

Powerlessness   The absence of power, whether imagined or real, is the expectancy that the behaviour of a person cannot determine the outcomes they seek.

Pressure group   Collective action to change the opinions and attitudes of society and to influence the policy-making process, for example, using lobbying, but not aiming to govern.

Protests (and demonstrations)   An expression of objection, by words or by actions, to particular events, policies or situations, that can take many different forms.

Protest song   Song to protest about perceived problems in society and to challenge the status quo by championing a cause.

Social movement   A sustained and organised public effort targeting authorities that can use both conventional and unconventional strategies to achieve its aims.

Soft power   The ability to obtain what one wants through indirect and long-term actions such as co-option and attraction.

Veganarchists   A philosophy of veganism and activism viewing the state as unnecessary and harmful to animals whilst observing a vegan diet.

Virtual sit-in   An activist tactic conducted entirely online by thousands of participants simultaneously to try to access a particular target website, rendering the server slow or collapsing it completely with the purpose of preventing others who want to visit the site from accessing it.

Bibliography

Abbott, S. and Killoran, A. (2005) *Mapping Public Health Networks*. London: Health Development Agency, published report.

Abel, G., Fitzgerald, L., and Brunton, C. (2007) *Report to the Prostitution Law Review Committee. The Impact of the Prostitution Reform Act on the Health and Safety Practices of Sex Workers*. Christchurch: University of Otago.

Abulof, U. (2011) 'What is the Arab third estate?' *The Huffington Post*, www.huffingtonpost.com/uriel-abulof/what-is-the-arab-third-es_b_832628.html, accessed 1 May 2011.

Adams, R.N. (1977) 'Power in human societies: a synthesis', in R.D. Fogelson and R.N. Adams (eds) *The Anthropology of Power: Ethnographic Studies from Asia, Oceania, and the New World*. New York: Academic Press, 387–410.

Aggleton, P. (1991) *Health*. London: Routledge.

Alinsky, S. (1971) *Rules for Radicals*. New York: Vintage Books.

Allmark, P., and Tod, A. (2006) 'How should public health professionals engage with lay epidemiology?', *Journal of Medical Ethics*, 32: 460–3.

Allsop, J., Jones, K., and Baggott, R. (2004) 'Health consumer groups in the UK: a new social movement', *Sociology of Health & Illness*, 26 (6): 737–56.

Alternative Press Center (2012) www.altpress.org, accessed 20 January 2012.

Altiok, Ö. (2007) 'Slow food movement', in G.L. Andersen and K.G. Herr (eds) *Encyclopedia of Activism and Social Justice*. London: Sage Publications.

Altogether Better (2011) 'York and Humberside public health observatory', www.yhpho.org.uk, accessed 23 May 2011.

Anderson, E. Shepard, M. and Salisbury, C. (2006) '"Taking off the suit": engaging the community in primary health care decision-making', *Health Expectations*, 9: 70–80.

Andersen, G.L. and Herr, K.G. (eds) (2007) *Encyclopedia of Activism and Social Justice*. London: Sage Publications.

Andrzejewski, J. R. (2007) 'Alternative press', in G.L. Andersen and K.G. Herr (eds) *Encyclopedia of Activism and Social Justice*. London: Sage Publications.

Appadurai, A. (2004) 'The capacity to aspire: culture and the terms of recognition', in V. Rao and M. Walton (eds) *Culture and Public Action*. California: Stanford University Press, Chapter 3.

ASH (2012) *Action on Smoking and Health*, www.ash.org, accessed 20 January 2012.

Avaaz (2012) www.avaaz.org, accessed 15 February 2012.

Ayaonline.org (2008) 'Scaling-up', www.ayaonline.org/Strategies/PDFs/ScalingUp.pdf, accessed 30 April 2008.

Ayers, M.D. and McCaughey, M. (2003) (eds) *Classifying Forms of Online Activism: The Case of Cyberprotests Against the World Bank in Cyberactivism: Online Activism in Theory and Practice*. New York: Routledge, pp. 72–73.

Baggott, R. (2000) *Public Health: Policy and Politics*. London: St. Martin's Press.

Baird, K.L., Davis, D.A. and Christensen, K. (2009) *Beyond Reproduction: Women's Health, Activism and Public Policy*. New York: Associated University Press.

Banks, K., Eagle, N., Rotich, J., Iyoha, C., Naidoo, A., Ngolobe, B.T., Kreutz, C., Reed, R., Atwood, A. and Ekine, S. (2010) *SMS Uprising: Mobile Activism in Africa*. Oxford: Fahamu Books and Pambazuka Press.

Barnes, M. (2002) 'User movements, community development and health promotion', in L. Adams, M. Amos and J. Munro (eds) *Promoting Health: Politics and Practice.* London: Sage Publications.

Barr, A. (1995) 'Empowering communities beyond fashionable rhetoric? Some reflections on Scottish experience', *Community Development Journal*, 30 (2): 121–32.

Barrig, M. (1990) 'Women and development in Peru: old models, new actors', *Community Development Journal*, 25 (4): 377–85.

Bassett, S.F., and Prapavessis, H. (2007) 'Home-based physical therapy intervention with adherence-enhancing strategies versus clinic based management for patients with ankle sprains', *Physical Therapy*, 87 (9): 1132–43.

Bassuk, E., Weinreb, L., Buckner, J., Browne, A., Salomon, A. and Bassuk, S. (1996) 'The characteristics and needs of sheltered homeless and low-income housed mothers', *Journal of the American Medical Association*, 276 (8): 640–6.

Baum, F. (2007) 'Cracking the nut of health equity: top down and bottom up pressure for action on the social determinants of health', *IUHPE Promotion and Education*, 14(2): 90–5.

Baum, F. (2008) 'The new public health', in *Oxford Higher Education*, 3rd edition. Oxford: Oxford Univeristy Press, p.704.

Baum, F. and Harris, E. (2006) 'Equity and the social determinants of health', *Health Promotion*, 17 (3): 163–5.

Bayoudh, F.S., Barrak, N., Ben Fredj, R., Allani, R. and Hamdi, M. (1995) 'Study of a custom in Somalia: the circumcision of girls', *Med Trop* (Mars), 55 (3): 238–42.

Benford, R.D. and Snow, D.A. (2000) 'Framing processes and social movements: an overview and assessment', *Annual Review of Sociology*, 26: 611–39.

Berkman, L. (1986) 'Social networks, support and health: taking the next step forward', *American Journal of Epidemiology*, 123: 559–61.

Bernier, N. (2007) 'Health promotion program resilience and policy trajectories: a comparison of three provinces', in M. O'Neill et al. (eds) *Health Promotion in Canada: Critical Perspectives.* Toronto: Canadian Scholars' Press Inc.

Berridge, V. (1999) 'Passive smoking and its pre-history in Britian: policy speaks to science?', *Social Science and Medicine*, 49: 1183–1196.

Berridge, V. (2007) 'Public health activism', *British Medical Journal*, 335: 1310–12.

Best, S. and Nocella II, A.J. (2006) *Igniting a Revolution: Voices in Defense of the Earth.* New York, A.K. Press.

Biddix, J.P. and Han Woo, P. (2008) 'Online networks of student protest: the case of the living wage campaign', *New Media and Society*, 10 (6): 871–91.

Big Issue (2012) www.bigissue.com, accessed 18 March 2012.

Bjaras, G., Haglund, B.J.A. and Rifkin, S. (1991) 'A new approach to community participation evaluation', *Health Promotion International*, 6 (3): 1999–2006.

Blair, D. and Bernard, J.R.L. (eds) (1998) *Macquarie Pocket Dictionary.* Sydney: Jacaranda Wiley Ltd.

Blood, R. (2011) 'Weblogs: a history and perspective', *Rebecca's Pocket*, www. rebeccablood.net/essays/weblog_history.html, accessed 12 July.

Bloor, M. and McIntosh, J. (1990) 'Surveillance and concealment', in S. Cunningham-Burley and N.P. McKeganey (eds) *Readings in Medical Sociology.* New York: Tavistock/Routledge.

Boethius, M.P. (2003) *The End of Prostitution in Sweden?* Stockholm: Swedish Institute.

Bopp, M., Germann, K., Bopp, J., Littlejohns, L.B. and Smith, N. (1999) *Evaluating Community Capacity for Change.* Calgary: Four Worlds Development.

Boseley, S. (2006) 'Herceptin costs "put other patients at risk"', *Guardian Weekly*, 8 December.

Boulle, J. and Avafia, T. (2005) 'Treatment Action Campaign (TAC) evaluation', www.tac.org.za/Documents/FinalTACEvaluation-AfaviaAndBoulle-20050701.pdf, accessed 2 August 2011.

Boutilier, M. (1993) *The Effectiveness of Community Action in Health Promotion: A Research Perspective.* Toronto: University of Toronto, ParticiACTION, p. 3.

Bracht, N. and Tsouros, A. (1990) 'Principles and strategies of effective community participation', *Health Promotion International*, 5 (3): 199–208.

Braithwaite, R.L., Bianchi, C. and Taylor, S.E. (1994) 'Ethnographic approach to community organisation and health empowerment', *Health Empowerment*, 21(3): 407–416.

Brashers, D.E., Haas, S.M., Neidig, J.L. and Rintamaki, L.S. (2002) 'Social activism, self-advocacy and coping with HIV illness', *Journal of Social and Personal Relationships*, 19 (1): 113–33.

Brashers, D.E. and Jackson, S.A. (1991) '"Politically savvy sick people": public penetration of the technical sphere', in D.W. Parson (ed.), *Argument in Controversy: Proceedings of the Seventh SCA/AFA Conference on Argumentation.* Annandale, VA: Speech Communication Association, pp. 284–8.

Braunack-Mayer, A. and Louise, J. (2008) 'The ethics of community empowerment: tensions in health promotion theory and practice', *Global Health Promotion*, 15 (3): 5–8.

Braveman, P. and Gruskin, S. (2003) 'Defining equity in health (theory and methods)', *Journal of Epidemiology & Community Health*, 57 (4): 254.

Brayne, H., Sargeant, L. and Brayne, C. (1998) 'Could boxing be banned? A legal and epidemiological perspective', *British Medical Journal*, 316: 1813–15.

Brian, D. (1997) *Animal Liberation and Social Revolution: A Vegan Perspective on Anarchism or An Anarchist Perspective on Veganism*, 3rd edition. Chicago: Firestarter Press.

Brown, V.A. (1992) 'Health care policies, health policies or policies for health?', in H. Gardner (ed.), *Health Policy Development, Implementation and Evaluation in Australia.* Melbourne: Churchill Livingstone.

Brown, P and Zavestoski, S. (2004) 'Social movements in health: an introduction', *Sociology of Health & Illness*, 26 (6): 679–94.

Brown, P., Zavestoski, S., McCormick, S., Mayer, B., Morello-Frosch, R., and Gasior, R. (2004) 'Embodied health movements: uncharted territory in social movement research', *Sociology of Health & Illness*, 26 (1): 50–80.

Brugger, N. (ed.) (2010) *Web History.* New York: Peter Lang Publishing.

Brunner, E. (1996) 'The social and biological basis of cardiovascular disease in office workers', in D. Blane, E. Brunner and R. Wilkinson (eds) *Health and Social Organisation: Towards a Health Policy for the 21st Century.* New York: Routledge.

Bryant, T. (2006) 'Politics, public policy and population health', in D. Raphael, T. Bryant and M. Rioux (eds) *Staying Alive: Critical Perspectives on Health, Illness, and Health Care.* Toronto: Canadian Scholars' Press.

Bullard, R.D. and Johnson, G.S. (2000) 'Environmental justice: grassroots activism and its impact on public policy decision making', *Journal of Social Sciences*, 56 (3): 555–78.

Burgess, R.G. (1982) *Field Research: A Source Book and Field Manual.* London: Allen & Unwin.

Burris, S. (1997) 'The invisibility of public health: population-level measures in a politics of market individualism', *American Journal of Public Health*, 87: 1607–1610.

Burton, B. (2007) *Inside Spin: The Dark Underbelly of the PR Industry.* Sydney: Allen & Unwin.

Byrne, P. (1988) *The Campaign for Nuclear Disarmament.* New York and London: Croom Helm.

Cakmak, C. (2007) 'Genital integrity activists', in G.L. Andersen and H.G. Kerr (eds) *Encyclopedia of Activism and Social Justice.* London: Sage Publications.

Campaign for Nuclear Disarmament (2012) www.cnduk.org, accessed 2 January 2012.

Cass, A., Lowell, A., Christie, M., Snelling, P.L., Flack, M., Marrnganyin, B. and Brown, I. (2002) 'Sharing the true stories: improving communication between Aboriginal patients and health care workers', *The Medical Journal of Australia,* 176 (10): 466–70.

Change (2012) www.change.org, accessed 15 February 2012.

Chapman, S. (1996) 'Civil disobedience and tobacco control: the case of BUGA UP. Billboard Utilizing Graffitists Against Unhealthy Promotions', *Tobacco Control,* 5: 179–85.

Charity Commission (2012) www.charitycommission.gov.uk, accessed 28 January 2012.

Chartered Institute of Environmental Health (2012) www.cieh.org, accessed 15 January 2012.

Chetwynd, J. (1996) 'The prostitutes collective: a uniquely New Zealand institution', In P. Davis (ed.), *Intimate Details and Vital Statistics: AIDS, Sexuality and the Social Order in New Zealand.* Auckland: Auckland University Press, pp. 137–47.

Chinn, D. (2011) 'Critical health literacy: a review and critical analysis', *Social Science and Medicine,* 73 (1): 60–7.

Christakis, N.A. and J.H. Fowler (2007) 'The spread of obesity in a large social network over 32 years', *New England Journal of Medicine,* 357(4): 370–9.

Clamshell Alliance (2012) www.clamshellalliance.org, accessed 21 January 2012.

Clarke, L. (Producer) and MacFarlane, K. (Director) (2005) *Prostitution: After the Act* (video tape). Wellington: Top Shelf Productions Limited. Available through New Zealand Film Archive, reference number: F88424.

Coban, A. and Yetis, M. (2007) 'Community-based ecological resistance movements', in G.L. Andersen and K.G. Herr (eds) *Encyclopedia of Activism and Social Justice.* London: Sage Publications.

Code Pink (2012) *Women for Peace,* www.codepink4peace.org, accessed 16 January 2012.

Cohen, D.R. and Henderson, J.B. (1991) *Health, Prevention and Economics.* Oxford. Oxford University Press.

Cohen, L., Baer, N. and Satterwhite, P. (1991) 'Developing effective coalitions: an eight step guide', in M.E. Wurzbach (ed.) *Community Health Education & Promotion: A Guide to Program Design and Evaluation,* 2nd edition. Gaithersburg, MD: Aspen Publishers Inc.

Cohen, R. (2007) 'Protest music', In G.L. Andersen and K.G. Herr (eds) *Encyclopedia of Activism and Social Justice.* London: Sage Publications.

Coleman, P.T. (2000) 'Power and conflict', in M. Deutsch and P.T. Coleman (eds) *The Handbook of Conflict Resolution: Theory and Practice.* San Francisco, CA: Jossey-Bass.

Collom, E. (2007) 'Home schooling', in G.L. Andersen and K.G. Herr (eds) *Encyclopedia of Activism and Social Justice.* London: Sage Publications.

Complete Computing (2012) www.complete.com, accessed 5 January 2012.

Confederation of British Industry (CBI) (2006) 'Transforming local services', Confederation of British Industry Brief. London, July 2006.

Cornish, F. (2006) 'Empowerment to participate: a case study of participation by Indian sex workers in HIV prevention', *Journal of Community and Applied Social Psychology,* 16: 301–15, DOI: 10.1002/casp.866.

Craig J. and Calhoun, C.J. (2002) *Classic Sociological Theory.* Oxford: Wiley-Blackwell.

Crosier, S. (2012) 'John Snow: the London Cholera epidemic of 1854', Center for Spatially Integrated Social Science, www.csiss.org/classics, accessed 14 May 2012.

Cwikel, J.G. (2006) *Social Epidemiology: Strategies for Public Health Activism.* New York: Columbia University Press.

Daly, S. (2007) 'Women's health activism', in G.L. Andersen and K.G. Herr (eds) *Encyclopedia of Activism and Social Justice.* London: Sage Publications.

Diamond J. (1997) *Guns, Germs and Steel: The Fates of Human Societies.* New York: W.W. Norton.

Diderichsen, F., Evans, T. and Whitehead, M. (2001) 'The social basis of disparities in health', in M. Whitehead et al. (eds) *Challenging Inequities in Health: From Ethics to Action.* New York: Oxford University Press.

Di Marco, G., Palomino, H., Altamirano, R., Mendez, S., and Palomino, M. de. (2003) *Movimientos sociales en la Argentina. Asambleas: La politización de la sociedad civil* (Social movements in Argentina. Meetings: The politicization of civil society). Buenos Aires, Argentina: Baudino Ediciones.

Dorkenoo, E. (1996) 'Combating female genital mutilation. An agenda for the next decade', *World Health Statistics,* 49 (2): 142–7.

Draper, P. (ed.) (1991) *Health through Public Policy.* London: Green Print.

Earle, L., Fozilhujaev, B., Tashbaeva, C. and Djamankulova, K. (2004) 'Community development in Kazakhstan, Kyrgyzstan and Uzbekistan'. Occasional Paper No. 40. Oxford: INTRAC.

Edirippulige, S., Marasinghe, R.B., Dissanayake, V.H.W., Abeykoon, P. and Wootton, R. (2009) 'Strategies to promote e-health and telemedicine activities in developing countries', in R. Wootton, N.G. Patil, R.E. Scott, and H. Kendall (eds) *Telehealth in the Developing World.* Ottawa, Canada: Royal Society of Medicine Press/IDRC.

Edwards, M., Howard, C. and Miller, R. (2001) *Social Policy, Public Policy: From Problem to Practice.* Sydney: Allen & Unwin.

EMCONET (2007) 'Employment conditions and health inequalities', *Final Report of the Employment Conditions Knowledge Network of the Commission on Social Determinants of Health.* Geneva: World Health Organization.

Emirbayer, M. and Goodwin, J. (1994) 'Network analysis, culture, and the problem of agency', *American Journal of Sociology,* 99: 1411–54.

Encyclopædia Britannica (2007) 'Animal rights: the modern animal rights movement', *Encyclopædia Britannica,* revised edition. London: Encyclopædia Britannica (UK) Ltd, p. 672.

Endresen, K. and von Kotze, A. (2005) 'Living while being alive: education and learning in the treatment action campaign', *International Journal of Lifelong Education,* 24: 431–41.

English, F.W. (2007) 'Alinsky, Saul (1909–1972)', in G.L. Andersen and K.G. Herr (eds) *Encyclopedia of Activism and Social Justice.* London: Sage Publications.

Everson, S.A., Lynch, J.W., Chesney, M.A., Kaplan, G.A., Goldberg, D.E., Shade, S.B., Cohen, R.D., Salonen, R. and Salonen, J.T. (1997) 'Interaction of workplace demands and cardiovascular reactivity in progression of carotid atherosclerosis: population based study', *British Medical Journal,* 314: 553–8.

Every Australian Counts (2012) http://everyaustraliancounts.com.au/, accessed 17 February 2012.

Eyerman, R. and Jamison, A. (1991) *Social Movements: A Cognitive Approach.* Cambridge: Polity Press.

Fathers4Justice (2012) www.fathers-4-justice.org, accessed 15 January 2012.

Faulkner, M. (2001) 'Empowerment and disempowerment: models of staff/patient interaction', *Nursing Times Research,* 6 (6): 936–48.

Fitzroy Legal Service Inc (2012) www.activistrights.org.au, accessed 18 February 2012.

Forman, L. (2007) 'Trade rules, intellectual property and the right to health', *Ethics and International Affairs*, 21 (3): 3–37.

Foucault, M. (1979) *Discipline and Punishment: The Birth of the Prison*. Harmondsworth, Middlesex: Peregrine Books.

Fox, S. and Rainie, L. (2001) 'Vital decisions: how internet users decide what information to trust when they or their loved ones are sick', in J. Hubley and J. Copeman (eds) *Practical Health Promotion*. Cambridge, UK: Polity Press, p. 182.

Francione, G.L. (1996) *Rain without Thunder: The Ideology of the Animal Rights Movement*. Philadelphia: Temple University Press.

Freeman, J. (ed.) (1983) *Social Movements of the Sixties and Seventies*. New York: Longman.

Freire, P. (1973) *Education for Critical Consciousness*. New York: Seabury Press.

Freudenberg, N. (1997) *Health Promotion in the City*. Atlanta: Centres for Disease Control and Prevention.

Freudenberg, N. (1978) 'Shaping the future of health education: from behaviour change to social change', *Health Education Monographs*, 6: 372–7.

Freudenberg, N., McDonough, J., and Tsui, E. (2011) 'Can a food justice movement improve nutrition and health? A case study of the emerging food movement in New York', *Journal of Urban Health*, 88 (4): 623–36.

Friedmann, J. (1992) *Empowerment: The Politics of Alternative Development*. Oxford: Blackwell Publishers.

Friedmann, S. and Motiar, S. (2005) 'A rewarding engagement? The treatment action campaign and the politics of HIV/AIDS', *Politics & Society*, 33: 511–65.

Frusciante, A.K. (2007) 'Leadership, participatory democratic', in G.L. Andersen and K.G. Herr (eds) (2007) *Encyclopedia of Activism and Social Justice*. London: Sage Publications.

Galer-Unti, R.A. (2009) 'Guerrilla advocacy: using aggressive marketing techniques for health policy change', *Health Promotion Practice*, 10 (3): 325–7.

Gallarotti, G. (2011) 'Soft power: what is it, why is it important and the conditions for its effective use', *Journal of Political Power*, 4 (1): 25–47.

Gangolli, L.V., Duggal, R. and Shukla, A. (eds) (2005) *Review of Health Care in India*. Mumbai: CEHAT.

Gasher, M., Hayes, M., Hackett, R., Gutstein, D., Ross, I. and Dunn, J. (2007) 'Spreading the news: social determinants of health reportage in Canadian newspapers', *Canadian Journal of Communication*, 32: 557–74.

Gauld, R. (2006) 'Health policy and the health system', in R. Miller (ed.) *New Zealand Government and Politics*. Auckland: Oxford University Press, p.525–35.

Gee, D. (2008) 'Park scheme seeks more "friends"', *The Christchurch Press*. www.bush.org.nz/library/934.html, accessed 3 April 2008.

GetUp! (2012) Action for Australia. www.getup.org.au, accessed 15 February 2012.

Gibbon, M., Labonte, R. and Laverack, G. (2002) 'Evaluating community capacity', *Health and Social Care in the Community*, 10 (6): 485–91.

Gibson, D. (2003) *Environmentalism: Ideology and Power*. New York: Nova Science Pub Inc.

Gillespie, D. and Melching, M. (2010) 'The transformative power of democracy and human rights in nonformal education: the case of Tostan', *Adult Education Querterly*, 60 (5): 477–98.

Glickman, L.B. (2009) *Buying Power: A History of Consumer Activism in America*. Chicago: University Of Chicago Press.

Goodman, R.M., Speers, M.A., McLeroy, K., Fawcett, S., Kegler, M., Parker, E., Rathgeb Smith, S., Sterling, T.D. and Grace, V.M. (1991) 'The marketing of empowerment and the construction of the health consumer: a critique of health promotion', *International Journal of Health Services*, 21 (2): 329–43.

Goodman, R.M., Speers, M.A., McLeroy, K., Fawcett, S., Kegler, M., Parker, E., Smith, S.R., Sterling, T.D. and Wallerstein, N. (1998) 'Identifying and defining the dimensions of community capacity to provide a basis for measurement', *Health Education & Behavior,* 25(3): 258–278.

Grace, V.M. (1991) 'The marketing of empowerment and the construction of the health consumer: a critique of health promotion', *International Journal of Health Services*, 21 (2): 329–43.

Granovetter, M. (1982) 'The strength of weak ties: a network theory revisited', in P. Marsden and N. Lin (eds) *Social Structure and Network Analysis.* Beverly Hills, CA: Sage Publications, pp. 105–30.

Gray, B. (1989) *Collaborating: Finding Common Ground for Multiparty Problems.* San Francisco: Jossey-Bass.

Greenpeace International (2012) Greenpeace International ww.greenpeace.org/, accessed 23 January 2012.

Hackett, M. (2007) 'Community radio and television', in G.L. Andersen and K.G. Herr (eds) *Encyclopedia of Activism and Social Justice.* London: Sage Publications.

Hager, N. (2009) 'Symposium on commercial sponsorship of psychiatrist education'. Speech to the Royal Australian and New Zealand College of Psychiatrists Conference, Rotorua, 16 October 2009.

Hann, S. and Wren, J. (2000) 'Decriminalisation', *Safety at Work*, 12 December, 7–9.

Haque, N. and Eng, B. (2011) 'Tackling inequity through a photo-voice project on the social determinants of health: translating photo-voice evidence to community action', *Global Health Promotion,* 18 (1): 16–19.

Harrison, J. (2007) *The Human Rights Impact of the World Trade Organisation.* Geneva: Hart Publishing.

Haynes, A.S., Gillespie, J.A., Derrick, G.E., Hall, W.D., Redman, S., Chapman, S. and Sturk, H. (2011) 'Galvanizers, guides, champions, and shields: the many ways that policymakers use public health researchers', *The Milbank Quarterly*, 89 (4): 564–98.

Haynes, A.W. and Singh, R.N. (1993) 'Helping families in developing countries: a model based on family empowerment and social justice', *Social Development Issues*, 15 (1): 27–37.

Hayward, B.M. (2006) *Public Participation in New Zealand Government and Politics.* Auckland: Oxford University Press.

Healy, C. (2006) 'Decriminalising our lives and our work: the New Zealand deal', in E. Cantin, J. Clamen, J. Lamoureux, N. Mensah, P. Robitaille, C. Thiboutot, L. Toupin, F. Tremblay (eds) Proceedings from Stella l'aime de maimie: eXXXpressions Forum Conference. Montreal: Stella, pp. 93–95.

Healy, C. and Reed, A. (1994) 'The healthy hooker', *New Internationalist*, 252, www.newint.org/issue252/healthy.htm, accessed 15 October 2008.

Ho, J. (2000) 'Self-empowerment and "professionalism": conversations with Taiwanese sex workers', *Inter-Asia Cultural Studies*, 1 (2): 283–99.

Hubley, J. and Copeman, J. (2008) *Practical Health Promotion.* Cambridge: Polity Press.

Hull, J. (1988) 'Not in my neighborhood'. Time (Time Inc), www.time.com/time/magazine/article/, accessed 25 January 2011.

Hunt, K. and Emslie, C. (2001) 'Commentary: the prevention paradox in lay epidemiology – Rose revisited', *International Journal of Epidemiology*, 30 (3): 442–6.

Iluyemi, A. (2009) 'Community-based health workers in developing countries and the role of m-health', in R. Wootton, N.G. Patil, R.E. Scott, and H. Kendall (eds) *Telehealth in the Developing World.* Ottawa, Canada: Royal Society of Medicine Press/IDRC.

Improvement Network (2011) www.tin.nhs.uk/patient-involvement, accessed 10 November 2011.

Independent Media Center (2012) www.indymedia.org, accessed 25 May 2012.

Israel, B.A., Checkoway, B., Schultz, A. and Zimmerman, M. (1994) 'Health education and community empowerment: conceptualizing and measuring perceptions of individual, organisational and community control', *Health Education Quarterly*, 21 (2): 149–70.

Jackson, T., Mitchell, S. and Wright, M. (1989) 'The community development continuum', *Community Health Studies*, 8 (1): 66–73.

Jerningan, D.H. and Wright, P. (1996) 'Media advocacy: lessons from community experiences', *Journal of Public Health Policy*, 17 (3): 306–30.

Jones, A. and Laverack, G. (2003) 'Building capable communities within a sustainable livelihoods approach: experiences from Central Asia', www.livelihoods.org/lessons/ Central Asia & Eastern Europe/SLLPC, accessed 1 September 2003.

Jones, L. and Sidell, M. (eds) (1997) *The Challenge of Promoting Health. Exploration and Action*. London: Macmillan.

Jones, L., Sidell, M. and Douglas, J. (eds) (2002) *The Challenge of Promoting Health: Exploration and Action*. London: Macmillan.

Kadushin, C. (1966) 'The friends and supporters of psychotherapy: on social circles in urban life', *American Sociological Review*, 31: 786.

Kant, I. (2004) *Kritik av det praktiska förnuftet* (Kritik der praktischen Vernunft). Stockholm: Thales.

Kashefi, E. and Mort, M. (2004) 'Grounded citizens' juries: a tool for health activism?', *Health Expectations*, 7 (4): 290–302.

Kasper, A. and Ferguson, S. (2001) *Breast Cancer: Society Shapes an Epidemic*, London: Palgrave Macmillan.

Kendall, S. (1998) (ed.) *Health and Empowerment: Research and Practice*. London: Arnold.

Kern, T. and Sang-hui, N. (2009) 'The making of a social movement. Citizen journalism in South Korea', *Current Sociology*, 57 (5): 637–60.

Khalaf, R. (2011) 'After the Arab Spring', *Financial Times*, 7 May: 1–2.

Kickbusch, I. (2002) 'The future of health promotion', http://info.med.yale.edu/eph/pdf/ The%20Future%20of%20Health%20Promotion.pdf, accessed 16 August 2011.

Kieffer, C.H. (1984) 'Citizen empowerment: a development perspective', *Prevention in Human Services*, 3: 9–36.

Kirigia, J.M., Seddoh, A. Gatwiri, A. Muthuri, L. and Seddoh, J. (2005) 'E-health: determinants, opportunities, challenges and the way forward for countries in the WHO African Region', *BMC Public Health*, 5: 137.

Kitzinger, J. (1995) 'Introducing focus groups', *British Medical Journal*, 311: 299–302.

Korsching, P.F. and Borich, T.O. (1997) 'Facilitating cluster communities: lessons from the Iowa experience', *Community Development Journal*, 32 (4): 342–53.

Klawiter, M. (2004) 'Breast cancer in two regimes: the impact of social movements on illness experience', *Sociology of Health & Illness*, 26 (6): 845–74.

Knudsen, T. (2007) 'Child labor laws', in G.L. Andersen and K.G. Herr (eds) *Encyclopedia of Activism and Social Justice*. London: Sage Publications.

KNUS (2007) 'Our cities, our health, our future: acting on social determinants for health equity in urban settings'. *Final Report of the Urban Settings Knowledge Network of the Commission on Social Determinants of Health*. Geneva: World Health Organization.

Kumpfer, K. Turner, C. Hopkins, R. and Librett, J. (1993) 'Leadership and team effectiveness in community coalitions for the prevention of alcohol and other drug abuse', Health education research', *Theory and Practice*, 8 (3): 359–374.

Krieger, N. and Birn, A. (1998) 'A vision of social justice as the foundation of public health: commemorating 150 years of the spirit of 1848', *American Journal of Public Health*, 88 (11): 1603–6.

Kroeker, C. (1995) 'Individual, organizational and societal empowerment: a study of the processes in a Nicaraguan agricultural cooperative', *American Journal of Community Psychology*, 23(5): 749–764.

Kumpfer, K., Turner, C., Hopkins, R. and Librett, J. (1993) 'Leadership and team effectiveness in community coalitions for the prevention of alcohol and other drug abuse', *Health Education Research: Theory and Practice*, 8(3): 359–374.

Labonté, R. (1990) 'Empowerment: notes on professional and community dimensions', *Canadian Review of Social Policy*, (26): 64–75.

Labonté, R. (1993) *Health Promotion and Empowerment: Practice Frameworks*. Toronto: Centre for Health Promotion/Participation.

Labonté, R. (1994) 'Health promotion and empowerment: reflections on professional practice', *Health Education Quarterly*, 21 (2): 253–68.

Labonté, R. (1996) 'Community development in the public health sector: the possibilities of an empowering relationship between the state and civil society', PhD thesis, York University, Toronto.

Labonté, R. (2000) 'Health promotion and the common good: towards a politics of practice', in D. Callahan (ed.) *Promoting Healthy Behaviour: How Much Freedom? Whose Responsibility?* Washington, DC: Georgetown University Press.

Labonté, R. and Laverack, G. (2001) 'Capacity building in health promotion, part 1: for whom? And for what purpose?', *Critical Public Health*, 11 (2): 111–28.

Labonté, R. and Laverack, G. (2008) *Health Promotion in Action: From Local to Global Empowerment*. London: Palgrave Macmillan.

Labonté, R. and Penfold, S. (1981) *Health Promotion Philosophy: From Victim-Blaming to Social Responsibility*. Vancouver: Health Promotion Directorate.

Labonté, R. and Schrecker, T. (2007) 'Globalization and social determinants of health: the role of the global marketplace (part 2 of 3)', *Globalization and Health*, 3, www. globalizationandhealth.com/content, accessed 22 June 2011.

Lancashire Public Health Network (2011) http://www.clph.net, accessed 12 January 2011.

Lasar, M. (2007) 'Media activism'. In G.L. Andersen and K.G. Herr (eds) *Encyclopedia of Activism and Social Justice*. London: Sage Publications.

Laverack, G. (1998) 'The concept of empowerment in a traditional Fijian context', *Journal of Community Health and Clinical Medicine for the Pacific*, 5 (1): 269.

Laverack, G. (1999) 'Addressing the contradiction between discourse and practice in health promotion', unpublished PhD thesis, Deakin University, Melbourne.

Laverack, G. (2001) 'An identification and interpretation of the organizational aspects of community empowerment', *Community Development Journal*, 36 (2): 40–52.

Laverack, G. (2004) *Health Promotion Practice: Power and Empowerment*. London: Sage Publications.

Laverack, G. (2005) *Public Health: Power, Empowerment and Professional Practice*. London: Palgrave Macmillan.

Laverack, G. (2006) 'Using a "domains" approach to build community empowerment', *Community Development Journal*, 41 (1): 4–12.

Laverack, G. (2007) *Health Promotion Practice: Building Empowered Communities*. London: Open University Press.

Laverack, G. (2008) 'The future of health promotion programming'. Workshop presentation 'Empowerment for health promotion: Global experiences, German perspectives', Munich, 21 January.

Laverack, G. (2009) *Public Health: Power, Empowerment & Professional Practice*, 2nd edition. London: Palgrave Macmillan.

Laverack, G. and Labonté, R. (2000) 'A planning framework for the accommodation of community empowerment goals within health promotion programming', *Health Policy and Planning*, 15 (3): 255–62.

Laverack, G. and Wallerstein, N. (2001) 'Measuring community empowerment: a fresh look at organizational domains', *Health Promotional International*, 16 (2): 179–85.

Laverack, G. and Whipple, A. (2010) 'The sirens' song of empowerment: a case study of health promotion and the New Zealand Prostitutes Collective', *Global Health Promotion*, 17 (1): 33–38.

Leiter, V. (2004) 'Parental activism, professional dominance, and early childhood disability', *Disability Studies Quarterly*, 24 (2).

Lerner, B.H. (2001) 'No shrinking violet: Rose Kushner and the rise of breast cancer activism', *Culture and Medicine*, 174: 362–5.

Lerner, M. (1986) *Surplus Powerlessness*. Oakland, CA: The Institute for Labour and Mental Health.

Lewis, D. (2003) 'Civil society', *Encyclopedia of Community*. London: Sage Publications, www.sage-ereference.com/view/community/n75.xml, accessed 5 December 2011.

Leyden, J. (2012) 'Hacker jailed for 32 months for attack on abortion-provider site', www.theregister.co.uk/2012/04/16/anon_jailed_over_abortion_site_hack/, accessed 20 May 2012.

Lichtenstein, B. (1999) 'Reframing 'Eve' in the AIDS era: the pursuit of legitimacy by New Zealand sex workers', in B. Dank and R. Refinetti (eds.) *Sex Work and Sex Workers: Sexuality and Culture*, vol. 2. New Brunswick: Transaction Publishers, pp. 37–59.

Lin, N. (2000) 'Inequality in social capital', *Contemporary Sociology*, 29: 785–95.

Linney, B. (1995) *Pictures, People and Power. People-Centred Visual Aids for Development*. London: Macmillan.

Linden, K. (1994) 'Health and empowerment', *The Journal of Applied Social Sciences*, 18(1): 33–40.

Lindquist, E.A. (2001) *Discerning Policy Influence: Framework for a Strategic Evaluation of IDRC-Supported Research*. www.idrc.ca/uploads/user-S/10359907080 discerning_policy.pdf

Lloyd, M. and Bor, R. (2004) *Communication Skills for Medicine*, 2nd edition. London: Churchill Livingstone.

London School of Economics (2006) *What is Civil Society?* www.lse.ac.uk/Depts/ccs/what_is_civil_society.htm

Loue, S., Lloyd, L.S. and O'Shea, D.J. (2003) *Community Health Advocacy*. New York: Kluwer Academic/Plenum Publishers.

Lupton, D. (1995) *The Imperative of Health: Public Health and the Regulated Body*. London: Sage Publications.

McCarthy, J.D. and Mayer N.Z. (1977) 'Resource mobilization and social movements: a partial theory', *American Journal of Sociology*, 82 (6): 1212–41.

McGrath, C. (2007a) 'Lobbying', in G.L. Andersen and K.G. Herr (eds) *Encyclopedia of Activism and Social Justice*. London: Sage Publications.

McGrath, C. (2007b) 'Coalition Building', in G.L. Andersen and K.G. Herr (eds) *Encyclopedia of Activism and Social Justice*. London: Sage Publications.

MacPherson, D.W. and Gushulak, B.D. (2004) *Global Migration Perspectives. Global Commission on International Migration*. Geneva: Report Number 7. Global Commission on International Migration.

Mackie, G. (1996) 'Ending footbinding and infibulation: a convention account', *American Sociological Review*, 61 (6): 999–1017.

Manandhar, D.S., Osrin, D., Prasad Shrestha, B., Mesko, N. Morrison, J. Tumbahanghe, K.M., Tamang, S., Thapa, S., Shrestha, D., Thapa, B., Shrestha, J.R., Wade, A., Standing, H., Manandhar, M.M., Costello, A., de L. and members of the MIRA Makwanpur trial team (2004) 'Effect of a participatory intervention with women's groups on birth outcomes in Nepal: cluster-randomised controlled trial', *The Lancet*, 364: 970–9.

MADD (2012) 'Mothers against drunk driving', www.madd.org, accessed 28 April 2012.

Marmot, M., Allen, J. and Goldblatt, P. (2010) 'A social movement, based on evidence, to reduce inequalities in health', *Social Science and Medicine,* 71: 1254–8.

Marsden, P. (2000) 'Social networks', in E.F. Borgatta and R.J.V. Montgomery (eds) *Encyclopedia of Sociology*, 2nd edition. New York: Macmillan, pp. 2727–35.

Marshall, G. (1998) *A Dictionary of Sociology*. Oxford: Oxford University Press.

Martin, B. (2007) 'Activism, social and political', in G.L. Andersen and K.G. Herr (eds) *Encyclopedia of Activism and Social Justice*. London: Sage Publications.

Marton cum Grafton (2012) Village website, http://marton-cum-grafton.org/oil_coop. htm, accessed 12 December 2011.

Mathieu, P.J. (2007) 'Homeless activism', in G.L. Andersen and K.G. Herr (eds) *Encyclopedia of Activism and Social Justice*. London: Sage Publications.

Mayeda, D., Chesney-Lind, M., and Koo, J. (2001) 'Talking story with Hawaii's youth: confronting violent and sexualized perceptions of ethnicity and gender', *Youth & Society*, 33 (1), 99–128.

Melucci, A. (1985) 'The symbolic challenge of contemporary movements', *Social Research*, 52 (4): 789–816.

Metoyer, A.B. (2007) 'Natural childbirth movement', in G.L. Andersen and K.G. Herr (eds) *Encyclopedia of Activism and Social Justice*. London: Sage Publications.

Micheletti, M. and Stolle, D. (2007) 'Mobilizing consumers to take responsibility for global social justice', *Annals of the American Academy of Political and Social Science*, 611: 157–75.

MindFreedom (2012) www.mindfreedom.org, accessed 21 March 2012.

Minkler, M. (ed.) (1997) *Community Organizing and Community Building for Health*. New Brunswick: Rutgers University Press.

Mirola, W.A. (2007a) 'Gay Liberation Front', in G.L. Andersen and K.G. Herr (eds) *Encyclopedia of Activism and Social Justice*. London: Sage Publications.

Mirola, W.A. (2007b) 'Eight-hour-day movement', in G.L. Andersen and K.G. Herr (eds) *Encyclopedia of Activism and Social Justice*. London: Sage Publications.

MissionMission (2012) www.missionmission.org, accessed 9 May 2012.

Mitchell, C. and Banks, M. (1998) *Handbook of Conflict Resolution. The Analytical Problem-Solving Approach*. London: Pinter.

Morozov, E. (2009) Moldova's twitter revolution, http://neteffect.foreignpolicy.com/posts/2009/04/07/moldovas_twitter_revolution, accessed 7 April 2011.

Morriss, P. (1987) *Power: A Philosophical Analysis*. New York: St. Martin's Press.

Mouy, B. and Barr, A. (2006) 'The social determinants of health: is there a role for health promotion foundations?', *Health Promotion Journal of Australia*, 17(3): 189–195.

Murguía, D. (2007a) 'Greenpeace', in G.L. Andersen and K.G. Herr (eds) *Encyclopedia of Activism and Social Justice*. London: Sage Publications.

Murguía, D. (2007b) 'Moore, Michael (1954–)', in G.L. Andersen and K.G. Herr (eds), *Encyclopedia of Activism and Social Justice*. London: Sage Publications.

Murray, S.A. and Graham, L.J.C. (1995) 'Practice based needs evaluation: use of four methods in a small neighbourhood', *British Medical Journal*, 310: 1443–8.

Nathanson, C. and Hopper, K. (2010) 'The Marmot review-social revolution by stealth', *Social Science and Medicine*, 71: 1237–9.

National Council on AIDS (1990) *The New Zealand Strategy on HIV/AIDS 1990*. Wellington, New Zealand: Department of Health.

National Heart Forum (2007) *Building Health. Creating and Enhancing Places for Healthy, Active Lives: Blueprint for Action*. London: UK National Heart Forum.

Navarro, V. (2009) 'What we mean by social determinants of health', *Global Health Promotion*, 16 (1): 5–16.

Navarro, V. and Shi, L. (2001) 'The political context of social inequalities and health', *Social Science and Medicine*, 52: 481–91.

Neilson, S. (2001) *IDRC-supported Research and its Influence on Public Policy. Knowledge Utilization and Public Policy Processes: A Literature Review*. IDRC Evaluation Unit. http://idrinfo.idrc.ca/archive/corpdocs/117145/litreview_e.html

Newkirk, I. (2000) *Free the Animals: The Story of the Animal Liberation Front*. New York: Lantern Books.

New Zealand Prostitutes Collective (NZPC) (2008) 'Our history', www.nzpc.org.nz, accessed 27 July 2011.

Nip, J. (2004) 'The queer sisters and its electronic bulletin board: a study of the internet for social movement mobilization', *Information, Communication & Society*, 7, 23–49.

Nomura, S. and Ishida, T. (2003) 'Computerized tools for promoting communities online', in K. Christensen and D. Levinson, *Encyclopedia of Community*. London: Sage Publications, www.sage-ereference.com/view/community/n362.xml, accessed 5 December 2011.

Nutbeam, D. (2000) 'Health literacy as a public health goal: a challenge for contemporary health education and communication strategies into the 21st century', *Health Promotion International*, 15 (3): 259–67.

O'Connor, M. and Parker, E. (1995) *Health Promotion: Principles and Practice in the Australian Context*. St Leonards, NSW: Allen & Unwin Pty Ltd.

Oneindia (2010) 'Indian American activists protest', http://news.oneindia.in, accessed 15 June 2010.

Onyx, J. and Benton, P. (1995) 'Empowerment and ageing: toward honoured place for crones and sages', in G. Craig and M. Mayo (eds) (1995) *Community Empowerment: A Reader in Participation and Development*. London: Zed Books, Chapter 5.

Pakulski, J. (1991) *Social Movements: The Politics of Moral Protest*. Sydney: Longman Cheshire.

Papa, M.J., Singhal, A. and Papa, W.H. (2006) *Organizing for Social Change: A Dialectic Journey of Theory and Praxis*. London: Sage Publications.

Parkinson, J. (2006) *Deliberating in the Real World: Problems of Legitimacy in Deliberative Democracy*. Oxford: Oxford University Press.

Patient Concern (2012) www.patientconcern.org.uk/, accessed 15 January 2012.

Patient UK (2012) www.patient.co.uk, accessed 21 May 2012.

Patients Association (2011) www.patients-association.com, accessed 15 December 2011.

Patterson, J. (2011) 'The Carlisle community center: designing for social capital in a small town', Lotus Development Corporation, IBM Watson Research Center.

Pearce, M. and Stewart, G. (2002) *British Political History, 1867–2001: Democracy and Decline*. London: Routledge.

Pearlin, L. and Aneshensel, C. (1986) 'Coping and social supports: their functions and applications', in D. Mechanic and L. H. Aiken (eds) *Applications of Social Science to Clinical Medicine and Health Policy.* New Brunswick, NJ: Rutgers University Press, pp. 417–37.

Peoples Health Movement (2012) www.phmovement.org, accessed 23 February 2012.

Perry, P. and Webster, A. (1999) *New Zealand Politics at the Turn of the Millennium.* Auckland: Alpha Publications.

Pescosolido, B.A. (1991) 'Illness careers and network ties: a conceptual model of utilization and compliance', in G. Albrecht and J. Levy (eds) *Advances in Medical Sociology.* Greenwich, CT: JAI Press, pp. 161–84.

Pescosolido, B.A. (1998) 'Beyond rational choice: the social dynamics of how people seek help', *American Journal of Sociology,* 97: 1096–138.

Pescosolido, B.A., Brooks-Gardner, C. and Lubell, K. (1998) 'How people get into mental health services: stories of choice, coercion and "muddling through" from "first-timers"', *Social Science and Medicine,* 46: 275–86.

Petrini, C. (2003) *Slow Food: The Case for Taste.* New York: Columbia University Press.

Photovoice (2008) 'Social change through photography', www.photovoice.com, accessed 5 March 2008.

Pimpare, S. (2007) 'Cloward, Richard A., and Piven, Frances Fox (1926–2001 and 1932–)', in G.L. Andersen and K.G. Herr (eds) *Encyclopedia of Activism and Social Justice.* London: Sage Publications.

Piven, F.F. and Cloward, R. (1977) *Poor Peoples' Movements: Why They Succeed, How they Fail.* New York: Pantheon Books.

Plows, A. (2007) 'Strategies and tactics in social movements', in G.L. Andersen and K.G. Herr (eds) *Encyclopedia of Activism and Social Justice.* London: Sage Publications.

Prostitution Law Review Committee (2008) *Report of the Prostitution Law Review Committee on the Operation of the Prostitution Reform Act 2003.* Wellington: Ministry of Justice, New Zealand Government.

Public Health Association of New Zealand (2001) 'Policy on decriminalisation of prostitution, www.pha.org.nz/policies/phapolicydecrimprostitution.pdf, accessed 22 July 2011.

Purdey, A.F., Adhikari, G.B., Robinson, S.A. and Cox, P.W. (1994) 'Participatory health development in rural Nepal: clarifying the process of community empowerment', *Health Education Quarterly,* 21 (3): 329–343.

Putnam, R.D. (1993) *Making Democracy Work: Civic Traditions in Modern Italy.* Princeton, NJ: Princeton University Press.

Putnam, R.D., Leonardi, R. and Nanetti, R.Y. (1993) *Making Democracy Work: Civic Traditions in Modern Italy.* Princeton, NJ: Princeton University Press.

Quandt, S.A. (2008) 'Food insecurity and hunger', in G.L. Andersen and K.G. Herr (eds) *Encyclopedia of Activism and Social Justice.* London: Sage Publications.

Rabinovitch, J. and Strega, S. (2004) 'The PEERS story: effective services sidestep the controversies', *Violence Against Women,* 10, 140–59, doi: 10.1177/1077801203260947.

Randall, S.I. (2007) 'Sanger, Margaret (1879–1966)', in G.L. Andersen and K.G. Herr (eds) *Encyclopedia of Activism and Social Justice.* London: Sage Publications.

Rappaport, J. (1984) *Studies in Empowerment: Steps toward Understanding and Action.* New York: Haworth Press.

Rappaport, J. (1987) 'Terms of empowerment/exemplars of prevention. Toward a theory of community psychology', *American Journal of Community Psychology,* 15: 121–47.

Rathgeber, E. (2009) 'Research partnerships in international health: capitalizing on opportunity'. Commissioned paper prepared for WHO-TDR meeting on research partnerships, Berlin, Germany.

Raven, B.H. and Litman-Adizes, T. (1986) 'Interpersonal influence and social power in health promotion', in W.B. Ward (ed.) *Advances in Health Education and Promotion*. London: Elsevier Science Ltd, pp. 181–209.

Reaves, J. (2007) 'Walking away from the past: how does an outsider change a culture? From the inside out says activist Molly Melching', *Chicago Tribune*. 25 November: 12.

Reber, B.H. and Kim, J.K. (2006) 'How activist groups use websites in media relations: evaluating online press rooms', *Journal of Public Relations Research*, 18(4): 313–33.

Rekart, M. (2005) 'Sex-work and harm reduction', *The Lancet*, 12: 2123–2135.

Renewal.net (2008) 'Resolving differences, building communities and Aik saath: conflict resolution peer group facilitators. Renewal.net case studies', www.renewal.net/Documents/RNET/, accessed 29 April 2011.

Renkert, S. and Nutbeam, D. (2001) 'Opportunities to improve maternal health literacy through antenatal education: an explanatory study', *Health Promotion International*, 16 (4): 381–8.

Richmond, R. (2002) 'Dr Alice Stewart: heroine of the anti-nuclear movement' (obituary), *British Medical Journal*, 325: 106.1

Rifkin, S.B. (1990) *Community Participation in Maternal and Child Health/Family Planning Programmes*. Geneva: World Health Organization.

Rifkin, S.B. (2011) 'Chasing the dragon: developing indicators for the assessment of community participation in health programmes'. Workshop presentation, 5 May. Ludwig Boltmann Institute for Health Promotion, Vienna, Austria.

Rifkin, S.B., Muller, F. and Bichmann, W. (1988) 'Primary health care: on measuring participation', *Social Science Medicine*, 9: 931–40.

Rifkin, S.B. and Pridmore, P. (2001) *Partners in Planning: Information, Participation and Empowerment*. Oxford: Macmillan Education.

Rissel, C. (1994) 'Empowerment: the holy grail of health promotion?' *Health Promotion International*, 9 (1): 39–47.

Roberts, A. (2009) 'Introduction', in A. Roberts and T. Garton Ash (eds) *Civil Resistance and Power Politics: The Experience of Non-violent Action from Gandhi to the Present*. New York: Oxford University Press.

Roberts, H. (1998) 'Empowering communities: the case of childhood accidents', in S. Kendall (ed.) *Health and Empowerment: Research and Practice*. London: Arnold, Chapter 6.

Robertson, A. and Minkler, M. (1994) 'New health promotion movement: a critical examination', *Health Education Quarterly*, 21 (3): 295–312.

Robson, C. (1993) *Real World Research*. Oxford: Blackwell.

Rohlinger, D.A. and Brown, J. (2009) 'Democracy, action and the internet after 9/11', *American Behavioural Scientist*, 53 (1): 133–50.

Rose, G. (1985) 'Sick individuals and sick populations', *International Journal of Epidemiology*, 14: 32–38.

Roughan, J.J. (1986) 'Village organization for development', PhD thesis, Department of Political Science, University of Hawaii, Honolulu.

Samuel, A.W. (2004) 'Hacktivism and the future of political participation'. PhD thesis, Department of Government, Harvard University, Cambridge, MA.

Saskatoon Regional Health Authority (SRHA) (2005) *Saskatoon 'In Motion': Five Years in the Making*. Saskatchewan: Saskatoon Regional Health Authority.

ScotPHN (2011) www.scotphn.net, accessed 15 December 2011.

Scrambler, G. (1987) 'Habermas and the power of medical expertise', in G. Scrambler (ed.) *Sociological Theory and Medical Sociology*. New York: Methuen Press.

Seedhouse, D. (1997) *Health Promotion: Philosophy, Prejudice and Practice*. New York/Toronto: Wiley & Sons.

Sen, A. (1999) *Development as Freedom*. New York: Alfred A Knopf Inc.

Seefeldt, F.M. (1985) 'Cultural considerations for evaluation consulting in the Egyptian context', in M.Q. Patton (ed.) *Culture and Evaluation*. San Francisco, CA: Jossey-Bass, pp. 69–78.

Seidman, S. and Wagner, D.G. (eds) (1992) *Postmodernism and Social Theory: The Debate Over General Theory*. Oxford: Blackwell.

Seligman, M. (1975) *Helplessness: On Depression, Development and Death*. San Francisco: W.H. Freeman.

Seligman, M. (1990) *Learned Optimism*. Toronto: Pocket Books.

Seligman, M. and Maier, S.F. (1967) 'Failure to escape traumatic shock', *Journal of Experimental Psychology*, 74: 1–9.

Serrano-Garcia, I. (1984) 'The illusion of empowerment: community development within a colonial context', in J. Rappaport (ed.) *Studies in Empowerment: Steps toward Understanding Action*. New York: Haworth Press, pp. 173–200.

Shadbolt, P. (2012) 'Sea Shepherd: whalers attack with grappling hooks', www.articles. cnn.com 18/1/2012, accessed 21 January 2012.

Shilts, R. (1982) *Mayor of Castro Street: The Life and Times of Harvey Milk*. New York: St. Martin's Press.

Silva, D.T., Uben, A.R., Wronski, I., Stronach, P. and Woods, M. (1998) 'Excessive rates of childhood mortality in the Northern Territory, 1985–94', *Journal of Paediatric Child Health*, 34: 63–8.

Small, C. (1999) 'Finding an invisible history', *Journal of Artificial Societies and Social Simulation*, 2: 3.

Smith, R. (2002) 'The discomfort of patient power', *British Medical Journal*, 324: 497–8.

Smithies, J. and Webster, G. (1998) *Community Involvement in Health*. Aldershot: Ashgate Publishing Ltd.

Speer, P. and Hughley, J. (1995) 'Community organising. an ecological route to empowerment and power', *American Journal of Community Psychology*, 23 (5): 729–48.

Starhawk, M.S. (1990) *Truth or Dare: Encounters with Power, Authority and Mystery*. New York: HarperCollins.

Statistics New Zealand (2007) 'QuickStats about culture and identity'. Wellington, www.stats.govt.nz/census/2006-census-data/quickstats-about-culture-identity/quickstats-about-culture-and-identity.htm, accessed 2 September 2008.

Stevenson, H. (2007) 'Guerrilla television', in G.L. Andersen and K.G. Herr (eds) *Encyclopedia of Activism and Social Justice*. London: Sage Publications.

Stewart, J., Kendall, E. and Coote, A. (1995) *Citizens' Juries*. London: Institute for Public Policy Research.

Stewart, M.A., Brown, J.B., Weston, W.W., McWhinney, I.R., McWilliam, C.L. and Freeman, T.R. (2003) *Patient Centred Medicine: Transforming the Clinical Method*, 2nd edition. Oxford: Radcliffe Medical Publications.

Stop Firestone (2012) www.StopFirestone.org, accessed 5 March 2012.

Strong, G. (1998) 'The gentle art of defeating a giant', *The Age*, Melbourne (21 November): 10.

Swift, C. and Levin, G. (1987) 'Empowerment: an emerging mental health technology', *Journal of Primary Prevention*, 8 (1 and 2): 71–94.

Syme, L. (1997) 'Individual vs community interventions in public health practice: some thoughts about a new approach', *Vichealth Letter*, July (2): 2–9.

Taylor, R. and Rieger, A. (1985) 'Medicine as social science: Rudolf Virchow on the typhus epidemic in Upper Silesia', *International Journal of Health Services*, 15(4): 547–59.

Tenbensel, T. and Davis, P. (2009) 'Public health sciences and policy in high income countries', in R. Detels, R. Beaglehole, M-A. Lansang and M. Guilford (eds) *Oxford Textbook of Public Health*. Oxford: Oxford University Press, pp. 796–809.

Tengland, P. (2007) 'Empowerment: a goal or a means for health promotion?', *Medicine, Health Care and Philosophy*, 10: 197–207.

Thangphet, S. (2006) 'Building capacity of community ecotourism for income generation and biodiversity conservation in Northern Thailand', Nagao Natural Environment Foundation, Chang Mai, Thailand.

Thomson, H., Petticrew, M. and Morrison, D. (2001) 'Health effects of housing improvement: systematic review of intervention studies', *British Medical Journal* (July), 323: 187–90.

Tilly, C. (2004) *Social Movements, 1768–2004*. Boulder, CO: Paradigm Press.

Toronto Department of Public Health (1991) 'Advocacy for basic health prerequisites: policy report', City of Toronto, Department of Public Health.

Tostan: Community Led Development (2011) 'Evaluations. The impact of the community empowerment program', www.tostan.org, accessed 2 October 2011.

Tracy, J.R. (2007) 'Housing movements', in G.L. Andersen and K.G. Herr (eds) *Encyclopedia of Activism and Social Justice*. London: Sage Publications.

Turner, B.S. and Samson, C. (1995) *Medical Power and Social Knowledge*. London: Sage Publications.

UK Animal Rights (2011) www.ukanimalrights.net, accessed 23 December 2011.

UNDP (2011) www.undp.org, accessed 15 December 2011.

UNICEF (2001) *Beyond Child Labour: Affirming Rights*. New York: UNICEF.

Uphoff, N. (1991) 'A field methodology for participatory self-education', *Community Development Journal*, 26 (4): 271–85.

Victurine, R. (2000) 'Building tourism excellence at the community level: capacity building for community-based entrepreneurs in Uganda', *Journal of Travel Research*, 38 (3): 221–9.

Vinthagen, S. (2007) 'Clamshell alliance', in G.L. Andersen and K.G. Herr (eds) *Encyclopedia of Activism and Social Justice*. London: Sage Publications.

Virtanen, M., Kivimaki, M., Joensuu, M., Elovainio, M., and Vahtera, J. (2005) 'Temporary employment and health: a review', *International Journal of Epidemiology*, 34 (3): 610–22.

Walker, K., MacBride, A. and Vachon, M. (1977) 'Social support networks and the crisis of bereavement', *Social Science and Medicine*, 11: 35–41.

Wallack, L.M., Dorfman, L., Jernigan, D. and Makani, T. (1993) *Media Advocacy and Public Health*. London: Sage Publications.

Wallerstein, N. (1998) 'Identifying and defining the dimensions of community capacity to provide a basis for measurement', *Health Education & Behavior*, 25 (3): 258–78.

Wallerstein, N. (1992) 'Powerlessness, empowerment and health. Implications for health promotion programs', *American Journal of Health Promotion*, 6 (3): 197–205.

Wallerstein, N. and Bernstein, E. (1988) 'Empowerment education: Freire's ideas adapted to health education', *Health Education Quarterly*, 15(4): 379–394.

Wallerstein, N. and Sanchez-Merki, V. (1994) 'Freirian praxis in health education: research results from an adolescent prevention program', *Health Education, Theory and Practice*, 9 (1): 105–18.

Walt, G. (1994) *Health Policy: An Introduction to Process and Power*. London: Zed Books.

Wang, C. and Burris, M. (1994) 'Empowerment through photo novella. Portraits of participants', *Health Education Quarterly*, 21 (2): 171–86.

Wang, C.C. and Pies, C.A. (2004) 'Family, maternal and child health through photovoice', *Maternal and Child Health Journal*, 8 (2): 95–102.

Wang, C., Yi, W.K., Tao, Z.W. and Carvano, K. (1998) 'Photovoice as a participatory health promotion strategy', *Health Promotion International*, 13(1): 75–86.

Wanless, D. (2003) *Securing Good Health for the Whole Population: Population Health Trends*. London: HMSO.

Ward, J. (1987) 'Community development with marginal people: the role of conflict', *Community Development Journal*, 22 (1): 18–21.

Wartenberg, T.E. (1990) *The Forms of Power: From Domination to Transformation*. Philadelphia, PA: Temple University Press.

Wasserman, S. and Faust. K.B. (1994) *Social Network Analysis: Methods and Applications*. New York: Cambridge University Press.

Weber, J. K. (2007) 'Virtual sit-ins', in G.L. Andersen and K.G. Herr (eds) *Encyclopedia of Activism and Social Justice*. London: Sage Publications.

Weber, M. (1947) *The Theory of Social and Economic Organization*. New York: The Free Press.

Welbourn, A. (1995) *Stepping Stones. A Training Package on HIV/AIDS, Communication and Relationship Skills*. London: ACTIONAID.

Werner, D. (1988) 'Empowerment and health', *Contact, Christian Medical Commission*, 102: 1–9.

Wheat, S. (1997) 'Banking on a better future', *Guardian Weekly*, 9 February: 19.

Whipple, A. (2008) 'The siren song of empowerment: a case study of the New Zealand Prostitutes Collective', MPH dissertation, School of Population Health, University of Auckland.

White, H.C. (1992) *Identity and Control: A Structured Theory of Social Action*. Princeton, NJ: Princeton University Press.

White, H.C., Boorman, S. and Brieger, R.L. (1976) 'Social structure from multiple networks, I. Blockmodels of roles and positions', *American Journal of Sociology*, 88 135–60.

Wilkinson, R. (1996) *Unhealthy Societies: The Afflictions of Inequality*. New York: Routledge.

Wilkinson, R.G. (ed.) (2003) *Social Determinants of Health: The Solid Facts*, 2nd edition. Copenhagen: WHO Regional Office for Europe.

Wilson, N., Dasho, S., Martin, A., Wallerstein, N., Wang, C., and Minkler, M. (2007) 'Engaging young adolescents in social action through photovoice: the Youth Empowerment Strategies (YES!) Project', *Journal of Early Adolescence*, 27 (2): 241–61.

World Health Organization (1948) Preamble to the Constitution of the World Health Organization as adopted by the International Health Conference, New York, 19–22 June.

World Health Organization (1978) *Declaration of Alma Ata*. Geneva: WHO.

World Health Organization (1986) *Ottawa Charter for Health Promotion*. Geneva: WHO.

World Health Organization (1998) *Health Promotion Glossary*. Geneva: WHO.

World Health Organization (2000) *Female Genital Mutilation*. Geneva: WHO.

World Health Organization (2005) 'The Bangkok Charter for health promotion in a globalized world', SixthGlobal Conference on Health Promotion. Bangkok: WHO.

World Health Organization (2007) 'Operationalising empowerment to improve maternal and newborn health: a guide to the workshop for maternal and newborn health programme managers and providers', Geneva: WHO (unpublished report).

World Health Organization (2008) 'Closing the gap in a generation'. Commission on Social Determinants of Health. Final Report. Geneva, WHO, www.who.int/social_determinants, accessed 6 May 2012.

Worsham, S. (2007) 'Code pink', in G.L. Andersen and K.G. Herr (eds) *Encyclopedia of Activism and Social Justice*. London: Sage Publications.

Wright, E.R. (1997) 'The impact of organizational factors on mental health professionals' involvement with families', *Psychiatric Services*, 48: 921–7.

Wrong, D.H. (1988) *Power: Its Forms, Bases and Uses*. Chicago, IL: University of Chicago Press.

Yeatman, A. (1998) *Activism and the Policy Process*. Sydney: Allen & Unwin.

Young, L. and Everitt, J. (2004) *Advocacy Groups*. Vancouver, BC: University of British Columbia Press.

Zakus, J.D.L. and Lysack, C.L. (1998) 'Revisiting community participation', *Health Policy and Planning*, 13 (1): 1–12.

Zimmerman, M.A. and Rappaport, J. (1988) 'Citizen participation, perceived control and psychological empowerment', *American Journal of Community Psychology*, 16 (5): 725–43.

Zoller, M.H. (2005) 'Health activism: communication theory and action for social change', *Communication Theory*, 15 (4): 341–64.

Index

NOTE: Page numbers in *italic type* refer to figures, figures in **bold type** refer to glossary entries.